Clinical Performance Data: A Guide to Interpretation

Margaret R. O'Leary, MD

JOINT COMMISSION

ON ACCREDITATION OF HEALTHCARE ORGANIZATIONS

Joint Commission Mission

The mission of the Joint Commission on Accreditation of Healthcare Organizations is to improve the quality of care provided to the public.

Joint Commission educational programs and publications support, but are separate from, the accreditation activities of the Joint Commission. Attendees at Joint Commission educational programs and purchasers of Joint Commission publications receive no special consideration or treatment in, or confidential information about, the accreditation process.

Printed in the U.S.A.   5 4 3 2 1

Requests for permission to reprint or make copies of any part of this book should be addressed to:
Permissions Editor
Joint Commission on Accreditation of Healthcare Organizations
One Renaissance Boulevard
Oakbrook Terrace, IL 60181

ISBN: 0-86688-434-3
Library of Congress Catalog Card Number: 95-77035

CONTENTS

FOREWORD

Water, water, everywhere,
Nor any drop to drink.
— Samuel Taylor Coleridge
  The Rime of the Ancient Mariner (1798)

As we approach the new millennium, we find ourselves awash in data...and at sea in understanding what all of these data mean.

Every day, individuals encounter data and, consciously or unconsciously, seek to convert the data into information. When the data are simple, familiar to the user, and of manageable scope, the conversion process—interpretation of the data—usually produces the correct information. Indeed, clinicians constantly use patient care data—symptoms, signs, and test results—in reaching usually correct diagnostic conclusions, and the meticulous translation of data that has been systematically collected through carefully designed research projects is the foundation for all advances in medical science.

However, data derived from measuring performance in health care—the performance of practitioners, provider organizations, and even community-based systems—are another story. In recent years, much excitement and enthusiasm have been generated by the rapid evolution of outcomes measures and other indices of performance. These new measurement tools have offered—and still do offer—the promise of a readily usable new source of information. However, these measures and the data they produce are not simple; they are anything but familiar to the user, and their scope is seemingly infinite.

In this information age, in which the demand for information continues to grow, and access to available information is now almost immediate, we in health care are not yet close to delivering on that promise. In fact, we must with some chagrin acknowledge the contentious, and thus far futile, dialogue that has evolved over the past decade:

The Public:	"We want the data."
The Providers:	"You can't have them."
The Public:	"We want the data. Give them to us.
The Providers:	"No. You won't understand the data.
The Public:	"Give us the data. We'll figure them out."
The Providers:	"OK. Here are the data."
The Public:	"You have to help us. We don't understand what the data mean."
The Providers:	"Neither do we."

Measurement enthusiasts, apparently poised in the recent past to spew forth a continuing stream of report cards, have missed an important step. What the public needs—indeed, what health care professionals need—is information, not raw data. What has been lost in the translation is the translation.

There is, nevertheless, an urgency to move forward. We must gain control over, understand, and translate health care performance data. Failing this, there will not only be no meaningful report cards, there will be no reliable foundation for outcomes management and other performance-improvement initiatives in health care. The array of existing information needs is impressive:

- Patients want performance information to help them choose among provider organizations and practitioners.
- Clinicians want performance information to help them improve the processes of care for specific conditions.
- Health care organization leaders want performance information to help them manage and improve their organizations' performance.
- Integrated delivery systems want performance information to help them select participating provider organizations and practitioners.
- Payers and purchasers want performance information to help them determine what to pay for and whom to pay.

- Public policy makers want performance information to help them ensure rational quality oversight requirements.
- Evaluators of health care organizations (such as accrediting bodies) want performance information to help them improve the value of their review activities.

Meeting these needs is what this book is all about. *Clinical Performance Data: A Guide to Interpretation* was written as a logical sequel to *The Measurement Mandate*, which emphasized the need for good data. This book is about producing good information, and it can certainly be read on its own.

Clinical Performance Data: A Guide to Interpretation invites health care professionals to take the lead in developing useful and accurate performance information. In so doing, it describes an explicit and rational approach to interpreting clinical performance data. Explicit, so that others can determine how interpretations of the data were undertaken—and whether they are reliable and valid. Rational, so that the interpretations are based on objective methods and logic, rather than potentially biased subjective judgments.

This explicit and rational approach to data interpretation is designed to help the reader answer the following questions:

- Which data can best be used to answer the question that has been posed?
- What have these data measured, and how did they measure it?
- How good are these data; what are their limitations?
- How can large volumes of data be summarized—and portrayed—in an understandable fashion?
- Is there variation in the data, and is this variation significant?
- What is the cause of the variation?

Almost all uses of performance data require an answer to this final question: Why are there differences in performance measurement data? Only by understanding the cause(s) of these differences can valid conclusions be drawn about performance. For example, if relatively high rates of morbidity or mortality following coronary artery bypass graft (CABG) procedures in one organization are caused by the relatively greater severity of illness of the patients who seek care there, decisions by the organization to change its procedures, or by patients to go elsewhere for care, are likely to be wrong.

But as important as the answer to the final question is, it is dependent on the answers to all of the preceding questions. Explicitly answering these questions provides the foundation for a rational answer to the final question—the one that counts. Just as using bad data can lead to bad decisions, so too can bad interpretation of good data. When we make decisions in the absence of data, we know we are guessing. When we make decisions based on bad data or bad interpretation of data, we are still guessing. But we may not know it.

This book is not simply a call for professional leadership in interpreting performance data. It urges healthy skepticism, critical thinking, and a splash of humility in approaching the final frontier of professional accountability to the public. The public does need to be educated about what the performance data mean, but we must first educate ourselves before we attempt to teach others.

The content of *The Measurement Mandate* and of *Clinical Performance Data: A Guide to Interpretation*—how to gather and interpret clinical performance data—is based on the Joint Commission's practical experience in developing both a contemporary framework for improving performance and a performance measurement system to support health care organizations in their improvement efforts. For both, we have drawn on the advice of many of the leading theoreticians and practitioners in the field, and have learned from the experiences of the many health care organizations that have sought accreditation, and those in particular who have participated in the developmental testing of the Joint Commission's Indicator Measurement System (IMSystem). This book builds off their advice and experience. We hope that readers will find it a valuable lifeline in the sea of data.

Dennis S. O'Leary, MD
President
Joint Commission on Accreditation
of Healthcare Organizations

CHAPTER ONE

Introduction to Clinical Performance Data Interpretation

L earning to interpret clinical performance data well is one of the most formidable challenges confronting health care providers today. *Interpretation is the multistep process by which meaning is assigned to raw clinical performance data.* Thus, interpretation is the process of making sense of, or understanding, data.

What, then, are clinical performance data? *Clinical performance data are neutral quantitative measurements of important patient care processes or patient health outcomes, generated by applying performance measures, commonly known as indicators.* Clinical performance data are both the output of performance measurement activities (described in other Joint Commission publications) and the input for the interpretation process described in this book.[1, 2] The position of clinical performance data in the performance improvement cycle is depicted in Figure 1 (see page 3).[3]

Examples of clinical performance data abound. For instance, the Joint Commission on Accreditation of Healthcare Organizations, in conjunction with hundreds of accredited hospitals throughout the United States, has gathered clinical performance data as part of the beta phase of its indicator testing process. Some of these data quantify important dimensions of clinical performance, such as effectiveness or timeliness, related to specified *patient care processes.* Dimensions of clinical performance and their definitions are listed in Table 1 (see page 4). Examples of clinical process measures include the following:

- Effectiveness with which organizations monitor the vital signs of seriously injured patients;*
- Appropriateness with which organizations use resources for patients with potential ischemic cardiac symptoms;†
- Effectiveness of preoperative diagnosis and staging for patients with lung cancer;‡ and
- Timeliness with which head-injured patients receive computerized tomography head scans.§

Other clinical performance data quantify *patient health outcomes.* Examples of clinical outcome measures include the following:

- Intrahospital mortality of patients undergoing isolated coronary artery bypass graft surgery or percutaneous transluminal coronary angioplasty, or with a principal diagnosis of acute myocardial infarction;** and

---

* The relevant Joint Commission Indicator Measurement System (IMSystem) indicator is: *Trauma patients with blood pressure, pulse rate, and respiratory rate documented on arrival to the emergency department and at least hourly for three hours, or until emergency department disposition, whichever is earlier.*
† The relevant Joint Commission IMSystem indicator is: *Patients admitted for acute myocardial infarction (AMI), rule-out AMI, or unstable angina who have a discharge diagnosis of AMI.*
‡ The relevant Joint Commission IMSystem indicator is: *Patients with nonsmall cell primary lung cancer undergoing thoracotomy with complete surgical resection of tumor.*
§ The relevant Joint Commission IMSystem indicator is: *Trauma patients with head computerized tomography (CT) scan performed: time from emergency department arrival to initial CT scan.*
** The relevant Joint Commission IMSystem indicator is: *Intrahospital mortality of cardiovascular patients undergoing isolated coronary artery bypass graft surgery, undergoing percutaneous transluminal coronary angioplasty, or with a principal diagnosis of acute myocardial infarction.*

FIGURE 1 Cycle for Improving Performance

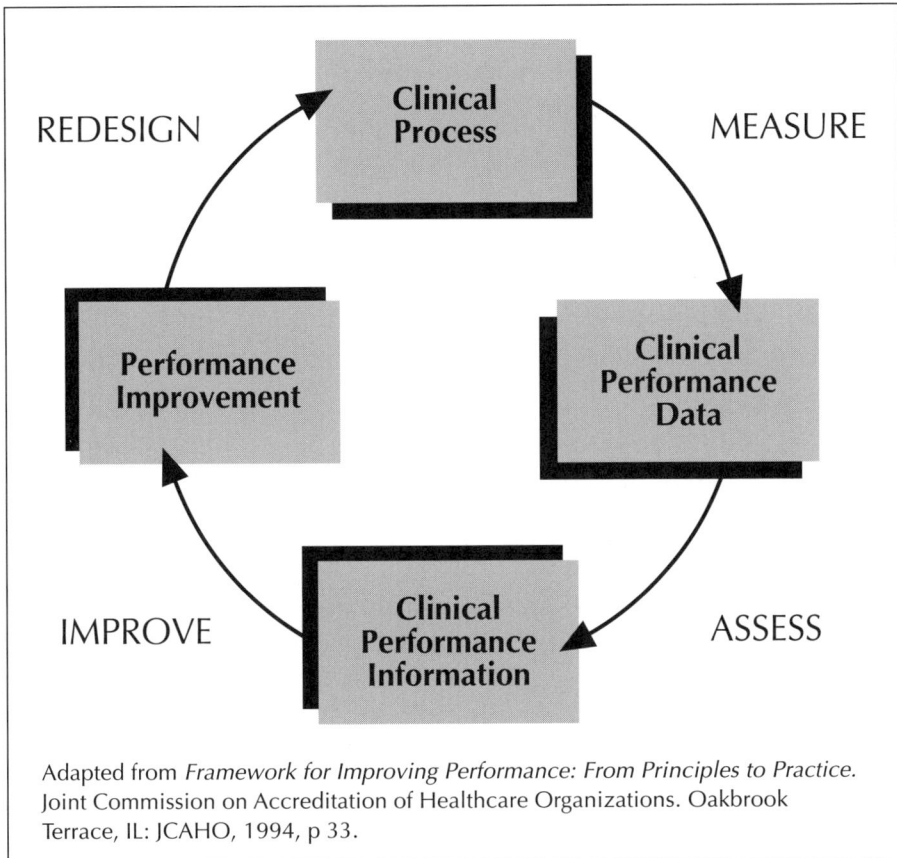

REDESIGN — **Clinical Process** — MEASURE

Performance Improvement

Clinical Performance Data

IMPROVE — **Clinical Performance Information** — ASSESS

Adapted from *Framework for Improving Performance: From Principles to Practice.* Joint Commission on Accreditation of Healthcare Organizations. Oakbrook Terrace, IL: JCAHO, 1994, p 33.

This cycle is composed of activities (represented by the arrows) and their related inputs and outputs (in boxes). The cycle is continuous and can be entered at any point.

- Intrahospital mortality of trauma patients with a systolic blood pressure of less than 70 mm Hg within two hours of emergency department arrival, who did not undergo a laparotomy or thoracotomy.*

---

* The relevant Joint Commission IMSystem indicator is: *Intrahospital mortality of trauma patients with a systolic blood pressure of less than 70 mm Hg within two hours of emergency department arrival, who did not undergo a laparotomy or thoracotomy.*

TABLE 1 Dimensions of Clinical Performance

Appropriateness
The degree to which the care/intervention provided is relevant to the patient's clinical needs, given the current state of knowledge

Availability
The degree to which the appropriate care/intervention is available to meet the needs of the patient served

Continuity
The degree to which the care/intervention for the patient is coordinated among practitioners, between organizations, and across time

Effectiveness
The degree to which the care/intervention is provided in the correct manner, given the current state of knowledge, in order to achieve the desired/projected outcome(s) for the patient

Efficacy
The degree to which the care/intervention used for the patient has been shown to accomplish the desired/projected outcome(s)

Efficiency
The ratio of the outcomes (results of care/intervention) for a patient to the resources used to deliver the care

Respect and Caring
The degree to which a patient, or designee, is involved in his or her own care decisions, and that those providing the services do so with sensitivity and respect for his or her needs and expectations and individual differences

Safety
The degree to which the risk of an intervention and the risk in the care environment are reduced for the patient and others, including the health care provider

Timeliness
The degree to which the care/intervention is provided to the patient at the time it is most beneficial or necessary

Source: Joint Commission on Accreditation of Healthcare Organizations: *The Measurement Mandate*. Oakbrook Terrace, IL: JCAHO, 1993, p 69.

Thesis of Interpretation

Interpretation operates on the thesis that *drawing accurate conclusions from raw clinical performance data depends on the degree to which the interpretive process is performed in an explicit and rational manner.* A conclusion is a judgment or decision reached after deliberation.

An *explicit* approach to interpretation is characterized by clearly developed, expressly stated, and carefully delineated tasks, such as the six tasks of interpretation described in Chapter Two. In contrast to explicit approaches, implicit approaches do not expressly state nor, in some cases, conceptualize distinct steps or tasks. Implicit approaches make it impossible for independent observers to determine exactly how conclusions are reached and whether these conclusions are reliable and valid.

A *rational* approach to interpretation is characterized by using informed reason, rather than emotion or personal prejudice, to form judgments. A rational approach to interpreting data is important because individual subjective, or intuitive, judgments tend to be biased and inaccurate.[4] It is well known in health care, for instance, that both providers and patients tend to overemphasize positive findings and ignore or underweigh evidence or data that contradict their initial beliefs. Among health care professionals, this bias does not appear to decrease with increasing expertise in a field.[4, 5] An interpretive approach must be rational *and* explicit because irrational ideas can sometimes be explicitly stated.

Benefits of a Formal Approach to Clinical Performance Data Interpretation

A formal approach to interpreting clinical performance data yields important benefits.

First, the reliability and validity of conclusions can be more effectively evaluated because the process by which these conclusions are drawn uses shared knowledge. People asked to use performance information, for example, can track backward through the interpretive steps to ask specific questions about how conclusions were reached. They might ask how the relevance of a certain process was determined, if at all, or they may have questions about the data's reliability.

Second, a formal interpretation process can establish a measure of accountability for conclusions reached by interpreters. Interpreters can be held accountable for conclusions they have drawn when the interpretive process they use is known. The ability to query interpreters is important today because "black box technology" is becoming increasingly prevalent. *Black box technology* refers to the use of an unknown clinical performance measurement system without understanding its inner workings.[6–8] Establishing a measure of accountability often has the added benefit of influencing interpreters who were previously indifferent to explicit and rational approaches to data interpretation. These interpreters often adopt a more rigorous approach to interpretation when they realize that their conclusions, and how they reached them, will be scrutinized.

Third, a formal approach to clinical performance data interpretation provides process overview and direction. This benefit is particularly useful to people who have limited experience in interpreting clinical performance data. The elements of interpretation and their interrelationships are clearly delineated, thereby providing boundaries and giving direction to the process. Discovering far downstream in the interpretation process that data lack integrity (say, reliability or relevance) will be less likely to occur when interpreters have a blueprint of the process to follow. This blueprint tells interpreters that evaluating data integrity should be performed early, rather than later, in the interpretative process.

Fourth, a formal approach focuses attention on clinical performance data interpretation as a complex cognitive process about which little is known. Conclusions about important matters, such as health, should, if possible, be backed by data and facts. How this "backing" process actually occurs, however, is only now being questioned. Extracting meaning from data is rarely simple.

Fifth, a formal approach provides a ready means for addressing the virtual avalanche of clinical performance data now beginning to reach the public domain. The current profusion of clinical performance data is the result of prodigious performance measurement efforts made by a variety of stakeholders, including state data commissions, the federal government, accrediting bodies, business coalitions, and entrepreneurial data organizations. In the past, providers, purchasers, public policymakers, and other groups interested in clinical performance data have assumed that making these data readily available would meet the health information needs of most groups. The growing consensus today, however, is that data by themselves are *not* sufficient; rather, they must be translated into information (that is, interpreted) to meet the information needs of various stakeholders.

The unmistakable reality for health professionals today is that they must rapidly learn the basics of clinical performance data interpretation. The learning curve may initially seem steep, but any initial difficulty is only temporary. The concepts and methods used to interpret clinical performance data are similar to clinical decision-making concepts and methods inculcated in clinicians during their training and reinforced throughout their professional careers. Clinicians, because of their health care backgrounds, are well suited to provide accurate and complete interpretations of clinical performance data. Their interpretations often become powerful stimuli for needed change and improvement in the delivery of health services.

Guiding Principles for Interpreters of Clinical Performance Data

There are several guiding principles for interpreters of clinical performance data.

First, interpreters must grasp the importance of their work. Data gain meaning and relevance only through their transformation into information. Information, not data, catalyzes change. The conclusions yielded by the interpretive process can influence decision making at many levels.

Second, interpreters must learn the importance of the different stages of data interpretation, including the order in which they occur. When all the stages of data interpretation are methodically carried out in the logical order, the accuracy and reliability of conclusions increase, and waste and rework are minimized.

Third, interpreters must be prepared to learn everything possible about the background, or context, of the clinical performance data being interpreted. The earlier that interpreters understand that data require a context to become meaningful, the more easily the interpretive process flows and yields better results. A bonus to becoming knowledgeable about the data's background is that data come alive, thereby reducing the tedium sometimes associated with working with data.

Fourth, interpreters should seek access to original data, especially if they are given data that have been manipulated or refined (for example, data summaries). Reviewing original data is beneficial for at least three reasons. First, many descriptive statistics, such as standard deviation or mean, summarize data to efficiently preserve the information contained in the individual measurements. Yet, in the process of summarizing data, some of the information contained in a collection of data is lost. Second, the deceptively simple act of reviewing original data gives interpreters a unique and personal understanding of data that cannot otherwise be achieved. Third, interpreters can judge the honesty and integrity of data suppliers by their willingness to share original data and explain the nature of manipulations that have been performed on the data.

Finally, interpreters should realize that data tend to be messy. An early appreciation that data do not always conform to a bell-shaped curve, but do come with some errors, can make the interpretation process more tolerable because the process is more predictable. Messy data are the rule, not the exception, in data interpretation. Interpreters must be wary of data that are flawless or otherwise too "clean."

Professional Attributes of Effective Interpreters

Cultivating certain professional attributes will improve interpreters' success in effectively translating clinical performance data into accurate and reliable performance information. First, interpreters should nurture their *problem-solving skills*, meaning the ability to work out correct solutions to questions and problems. The interpretation process often poses challenges, such as how to approach data that possess a low level of reliability or do not conform (or conform too well) to a bell-shaped curve.

Effective interpreters work at being as *thorough* as possible, meaning that they are painstakingly careful in assessing performance data. Many operations are performed on data throughout the interpretation process; a mistake made during the process can have subsequent, sometimes serious, undesirable effects. Thorough interpreters actively look for and usually find their mistakes before they cause waste or harm.

Open-mindedness is an important quality of good interpreters. Open-mindedness means receptiveness to new and different ideas or the opinions of others. There are sufficient challenges in ushering data through the interpretation process to make new and different ideas and opinions not only welcome but necessary.

Awareness of one's own limitations is an important professional attribute of interpreters. Since mistakes are unavoidable over time, effective interpreters know when to ask for assistance.

Effective interpreters should develop a *healthy degree of skepticism*, meaning a questioning attitude and state of mind. There are few manipulations or results of performance data interpretation that should *not* be questioned. Questioning improves understanding and learning and increases the probability that errors and omissions will be detected.

The ability to *collaborate* is an essential trait of an effective interpreter. Collaborate, in this context, means the ability to work in a joint intellectual effort with other professionals who are involved in the interpretation process. For instance, data or information specialists responsible for creating performance data reports for clinicians should have skill in collaborating with clinicians so that the reports adequately meet the clinicians' needs.

Interpreters must strive to exchange ideas effectively, that is, *communicate* well with other people, both orally and in writing. Effective communication is particularly important because the success or failure of interpretation depends on the ability of interpreters to lead other people to a personal "discovery" of performance improvement opportunities. Poorly designed graphs, tables containing too much data, a dearth of explanatory text to accompany visual or numerical descriptions of data, and an arrogant demeanor are some examples of poor communication that can thwart an entire performance improvement function.

Interpreters must be able to think and express themselves in quantitative terms (*numeracy*).[9] It is virtually impossible to avoid numbers during the process of interpreting clinical performance data. Data interpretation depends on the effective handling and manipulation of numbers. People who lack mathematical understanding will likely experience considerable frustration. "Numerate" interpreters invariably strengthen performance data interpretation.

Finally, effective interpreters attain a degree of *computer literacy*, meaning that they learn to operate a computer and understand the software used for storing, retrieving, and manipulating clinical performance data. Computer support has become essential for performance database development and application.

Summary Observations

Clinical performance data interpretation is a new challenge for many health care professionals because of unfamiliarity with clinical performance data and interpretive techniques and the rapidity with which data requiring interpretation are reaching the public domain. This chapter outlines six important points that set the stage for presenting the formal (explicit and rational) approach to clinical performance data interpretation described in Chapter Two.

1. Clinical performance data interpretation is the process of assigning meaning to, or making sense of, raw data.

2. Clinical performance data are neutral quantitative measurements of important patient care processes or patient health outcomes, generated by applying performance measures, known as indicators.

3. Clinical performance data interpretation operates on the thesis that drawing accurate and reliable conclusions from raw performance data depends on the degree to which the interpretive process is performed in an explicit and rational, or formal, manner.

4. A formal approach to clinical performance data interpretation yields several important benefits, including improving evaluation of performance conclusions; enhancing accountability for conclusions; providing process overview and direction; understanding that data interpretation is a complex, relatively unstudied, cognitive process; and providing a ready means for addressing clinical performance data now beginning to reach the public domain.

5. Guiding principles for interpreters of clinical performance data are grasping the importance of the process they are undertaking; learning the importance of the different stages of data interpretation, including the order in which they occur; studying the characteristics and attributes of clinical performance data; seeking access to original data for personal review; and understanding that data tend to be messy.

6. Professional attributes of effective interpreters include problem-solving skills, thoroughness, open-mindedness, awareness of one's own limitations, a healthy degree of skepticism, the ability to collaborate with other people, communication skills, numeracy, and computer literacy.

References

1.   Joint Commission on Accreditation of Healthcare Organizations: *Primer on Indicator Development and Application.* Oakbrook Terrace, IL: JCAHO, 1990.

2.   Joint Commission on Accreditation of Healthcare Organizations: *The Measurement Mandate.* Oakbrook Terrace, IL: JCAHO, 1993.

3.   Joint Commission on Accreditation of Healthcare Organizations: *Framework for Improving Performance: From Principles to Practice.* Oakbrook Terrace, IL: JCAHO, 1994.

4.   Chow CW, Haddad KM, Wong-Boren A: Improving subjective decision making in health care administration. *Hospital and Health Services Administration* 36:191–211, 1991.

5.   Elstein AS, Shulman LS, Sprafka SA: *Medical Problem Solving: An Analysis of Clinical Reasoning.* Cambridge: Cambridge University Press, 1978.

6.   Joint Commission on Accreditation of Healthcare Organizations: *The Measurement Mandate.* Oakbrook Terrace, IL: JCAHO, 1993, pp v–ix.

7.   Iezzoni LI: "Black box" medical information systems: A technology needing assessment. *JAMA* 265:3006–3007, 1991.

8.   Blumberg MS: Biased estimates of expected acute myocardial infarction mortality using MedisGroups admission severity groups. *JAMA* 265:2965–2970, 1991.

9.   Paulos JA: *Innumeracy: Mathematical Illiteracy and Its Consequences.* New York: Random House, 1990.

CHAPTER TWO

Overview of the
Elements of Interpretation

S ix tasks form the explicit and rational approach to clinical performance interpretation described in this book:
- Select a specific interpretation focus;
- Study characteristics of clinical performance data;
- Evaluate the strength of the data;
- Summarize the data;
- Study variation to identify undesirable variation; and
- Determine underlying causes of undesirable variation.

A brief overview of each interpretive task introduces the subsequent chapters. Each task is analyzed using the experiences gained and lessons learned by the Joint Commission and participating health care organizations during the early stages of Joint Commission indicator data analysis and interpretation activities.

First Interpretive Task:
Select a Specific Interpretation Focus

Specificity is a prerequisite for successful interpretation efforts. Interpreters must demonstrate restraint, at least initially, by narrowing the scope of their interpretation efforts to a workable amount of focused data. A useful unit of data for interpretation is an indicator-specific data set or, simply, indicator data set. *An indicator data set is a collection of data generated by a single indicator.* A single indicator data set would be, for example, the data generated by applying the indicator that measures the timeliness with which an organization provides surgical procedures for its trauma patients with selected injuries, such as liver or spleen laceration.* Selecting a specific interpretation focus is discussed in detail in Chapter Three.

Second Interpretive Task: Study Characteristics of Clinical Performance Data

Raw performance data do not possess intrinsic meaning; rather, each indicator data set has (or should have) corresponding indicator information, which is sometimes called an *indicator information set.* An indicator information set typically includes:

- an indicator statement;
- definition of terms;
- the indicator type;
- a rationale;
- a description of the indicator population;
- indicator data collection logic;
- underlying factors that may explain variations in data.

An indicator information set gives users a context for, and important characteristics of, the data.[1]

Important characteristics of data include whether they measure a desirable or an undesirable process or outcome, express information about many events or about individual events, and express information as a continuous variable or a discrete variable. Examples of indicator information sets are given in Figure 2 (Joint Commission beta indicator; see pages 16–20) and Figure 3 (IMSystem indicator; see pages 22–28). Characteristics of clinical performance data are described in detail in Chapter Four.

---

* The relevant Joint Commission IMSystem indicator is: *Trauma patients undergoing selected neurosurgical, orthopedic, or abdominal surgical procedures: time from emergency department arrival to procedure.*

Third Interpretive Task:
Evaluate the Strength of the Data

As described in Chapter Five, the strength of data is judged by six standards:

- their clinical relevance to multiple stakeholders;
- the range of health care processes and outcomes that they address;
- their degree of reliability;
- their degree of validity;
- their degree of variation; and
- how much control health care providers have over the process or outcome measured by the data.

The third task of interpretation is critical for judging whether data possess sufficient strength to warrant continuing the interpretive process. If they do not, interpreters must decide whether the data can be salvaged.

Fourth Interpretive Task:
Summarize the Data

Clinical performance data must be expressed in a simple form that will permit conclusions to be drawn, either directly or through further calculations. A long list of cardiovascular cases that meet the criteria for a particular indicator event is not particularly helpful (beyond providing material for interested persons to work on) because it is impossible to detect important relationships from the unsorted mass of raw material.[2]

One way of sorting raw material is to construct a frequency distribution by tabulating indicator-specific measurements, such as indicator-specific rates for 1,000 hospitals. Certain values must then be calculated to describe the characteristics of that frequency distribution. These values permit comparisons between one series of observations and another. As described in detail in Chapter Six, two principal characteristics of the frequency distribution must be quantified: its *location* and *spread*. *Location* (also

FIGURE 2 Indicator Information Set for Beta Indicator TR-12

TR-12 Indicator Focus: Systems necessary for obtaining autopsies for trauma victims.

I. Indicator (Numerator)
Trauma patients who died within 48 hours of emergency department (ED) arrival for whom an autopsy was performed.

II. Definition of Terms
(Indicator terms that may be ambiguous or need further explanation for collection purposes.)

Autopsy: Postmortem examination of internal organs and brain by pathologist.

ED Arrival: Ambulance arrival time at the initial receiving acute care facility or, if not transported by ambulance, first documented ED time.

III. Type of Indicator
A. This is a:
   /   / sentinel event indicator (all occurrences warrant investigation);
   or
   /✔/ rate-based indicator (further assessment warranted if the occurrence rate shows a significant trend, exceeds predetermined thresholds, or indicates significant differences when compared to peer institutions).
B. This indicator primarily addresses:
   /✔/ a process of patient care;
   or
   /   / a patient outcome.

The Joint Commission Trauma Care Task Force for Indicator Development developed this indicator information set to help interpret data collected for Beta Indicator TR-12 (*trauma patients who expired within 48 hours of emergency department arrival for whom an autopsy was performed*).

FIGURE 2 (Continued)

IV. Rationale

A. Intent of monitoring the indicator event:

The autopsy process yields valuable information on clinical practices that may have contributed to patient death. Although there is significant regional variation in terms of coroner and medical examiner aggressiveness in determining cause of death for trauma patients, the rate of autopsies for a given hospital may indicate the medical staff's commitment to understanding the cause of death and improving overall quality of care. Low rates in comparison to peer institutions would signal the need for in-depth evaluation.

B. Selected references:

American College of Surgeons, Committee on Trauma: Hospital and prehospital resources for optimal care of the injured patient. *Bulletin of the ACS*; Appendix G: No. 1.

C. The components of patient care assessed by this indicator:

1. Medical staff commitment to understanding trauma deaths.

2. Regional commitment to understanding trauma deaths.

V. Description of Indicator Population

A. Subcategories (patient subpopulations by which the indicator data will be separated for analysis):

None

B. Indicator data format (the manner in which indicator data will be expressed):

1. Rate-based indicator format:

a. Numerator(s): Number of trauma patients undergoing autopsy who die within 48 hours of ED arrival.

b. Denominator(s): Number of trauma patients who die within 48 hours of ED arrival.

2. Sentinel event indicator format: N/A

Continued on next page

FIGURE 2 Indicator Information Set for Beta Indicator TR-12 (Continued)

VI. Indicator Logic   **TR-12:** Trauma patients who expired within 48 hours of emergency department (ED) arrival for whom an autopsy was performed

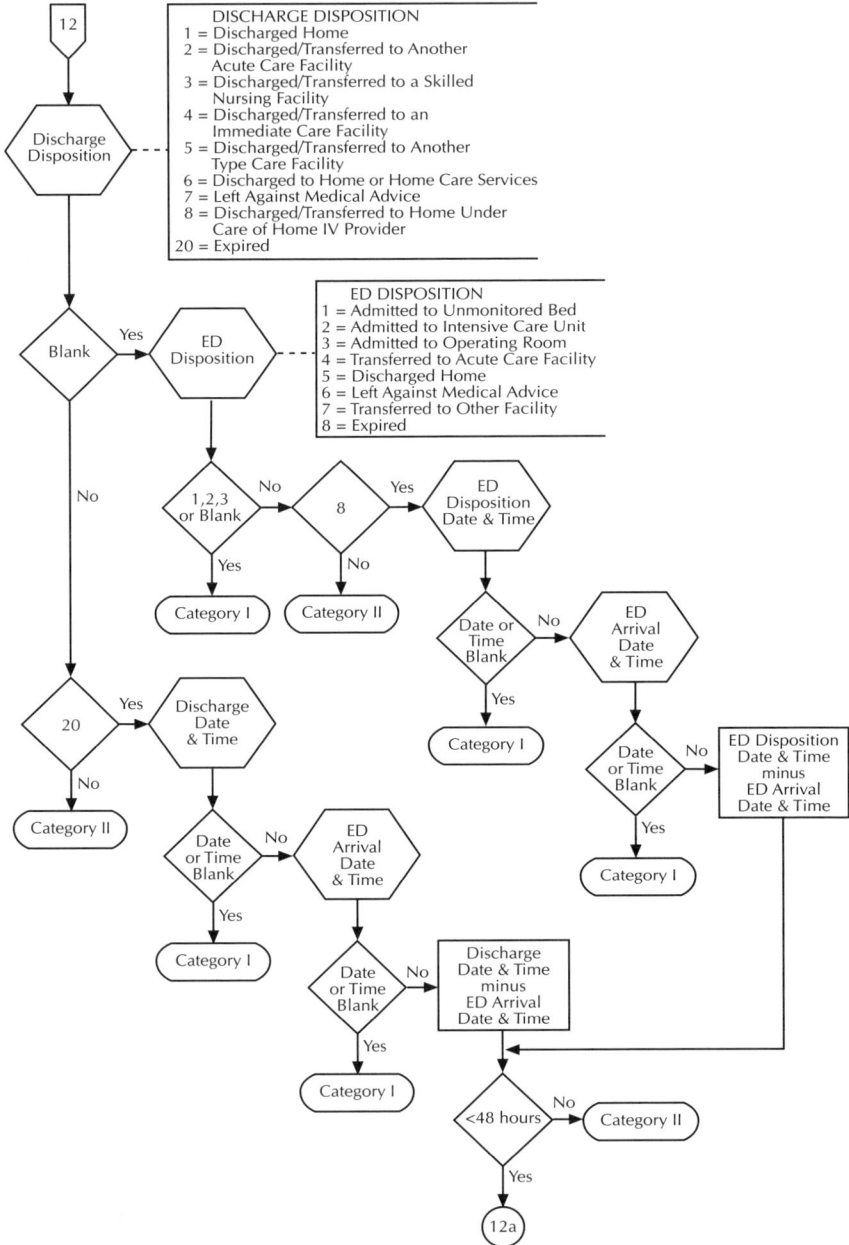

DISCHARGE DISPOSITION
1 = Discharged Home
2 = Discharged/Transferred to Another Acute Care Facility
3 = Discharged/Transferred to a Skilled Nursing Facility
4 = Discharged/Transferred to an Immediate Care Facility
5 = Discharged/Transferred to Another Type Care Facility
6 = Discharged to Home or Home Care Services
7 = Left Against Medical Advice
8 = Discharged/Transferred to Home Under Care of Home IV Provider
20 = Expired

ED DISPOSITION
1 = Admitted to Unmonitored Bed
2 = Admitted to Intensive Care Unit
3 = Admitted to Operating Room
4 = Transferred to Acute Care Facility
5 = Discharged Home
6 = Left Against Medical Advice
7 = Transferred to Other Facility
8 = Expired

Continued on next page

FIGURE 2 (Continued)

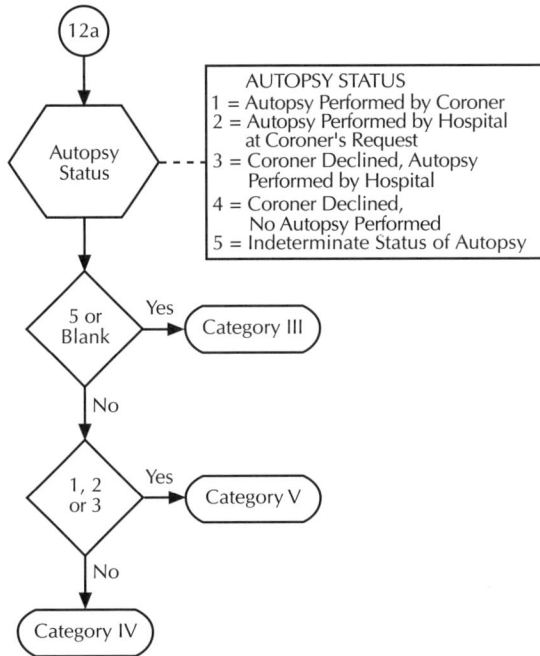

AUTOPSY STATUS
1 = Autopsy Performed by Coroner
2 = Autopsy Performed by Hospital
    at Coroner's Request
3 = Coroner Declined, Autopsy
    Performed by Hospital
4 = Coroner Declined,
    No Autopsy Performed
5 = Indeterminate Status of Autopsy

VII. Underlying Factors

Factors not included in the indicator that may account for significant indicator rates or indicator activity:

A. Patient-based factors (factors outside the health care
organization's control contributing to patient outcomes)

1. Severity of illness (factors related to the degree or stage of
disease before treatment);

2. Comorbid conditions (disease factors, not intrinsic to the
primary disease, which may have an impact on patient suitability
for, or tolerance of, diagnostic or therapeutic care); or

3. Other patient factors (nondisease factors that may have an
impact on care, such as age, sex, refusal of consent):

a. refusal to consent by patient's family,

Continued on next page

FIGURE 2 Indicator Information Set for Beta Indicator TR-12 (Continued)

> b. inadequate staffing of coroner's or medical examiner's office, or
>
> c. determination by coroner or medical examiner that autopsy would yield no additional information on cause of death.
>
> B. Nonpatient-based factors:
>
> 1. Practitioner-based factors (factors related to specific health care practitioners, for example, physicians, nurses, respiratory therapists):
>
>> a. failure of physicians to request autopsy
>
> 2. Organization-based factors (factors related to the health care organization that contribute to either specific aspects of patient care or to the general ability of direct caregivers to provide services):
>
>> a. fear of malpractice litigation,
>>
>> b. inadequate staffing of coroner's or medical examiner's office,
>>
>> c. jurisdictional confusion, or
>>
>> d. failure to inform coroner or medical examiner of death.
>
> **Source:** *Joint Commission on Accreditation of Healthcare Organizations Trauma, Oncology, and Cardiovascular Indicators Beta Phase Training Manual and Software User's Guide,* 1991.

called central tendency or average value) is a measure of the position of the distribution—that is, the point around which the individual values are dispersed. *Spread* (also called dispersion or scatter) of the observations is a measure of their scatter around an average value.

In practice, it is constantly necessary to discuss and compare measures of central tendency and dispersion. When two distributions differ in their location, their spread, or both, interpreters are led to seek the reasons for the difference. Numerical descriptions of frequency distributions of data are often augmented with visual descriptions of data, such as control charts.

Fifth Interpretive Task: Identify Undesirable Data Variation

Variation is fluctuation in a series of results. A certain amount of variation is the inevitable product (output) of any system or process. Unusual variation is a departure from this steady state. Unusual variation may be desirable (for example, a marked reduction in primary cesarean section rates) or undesirable (a marked increase in nosocomial infection rates). Undesirable variation concerns health care organizations more because it consumes organization time and resources and does not typically contribute to the creation of value.[3] Thus, the immediate goal of studying variation is to identify the occurrence of *unusual, undesirable* variation in data.

Unusual variation is not always easy to recognize. Indeed, variation tends to create confusion among human beings.[4] To address this circumstance, Dr Walter Shewhart developed a technique to study variation by making a distinction between stable variation and unstable variation in a series of results.[5–7] He devised the *control chart* to provide a consistent method to study variation *within processes over time*, and to link variation to its causes (common causes of stable variation versus special causes of unstable variation). The control chart and its rules for use allow interpreters to make clear and repeatable judgments of the state of statistical control of variation in the results (see Figure 4, page 30).

A *comparison chart* is a second analytic tool that is used to study variation *across different organizations* (see Figure 5, page 31). In comparison charts, the data must be risk-adjusted for patient characteristics over which the health care organization has no control, such as patient age. This adjustment permits observed differences between one organization and another to be attributed to nonpatient-based factors, rather than differences in the patient populations treated by the different institutions. Studying variation is described fully in Chapter Seven.

FIGURE 3 Indicator Information Set for IMSystem Indicator 22

Focus: Airway management of comatose trauma patients

Indicator Statement

Numerator—Comatose trauma patients with selected intracranial injuries discharged from the emergency department (ED) prior to endotracheal intubation or cricothyrotomy.

Denominator—Emergency department comatose trauma patients with selected intracranial injuries.

Subcategories—None

Indicator Objectives and Suggested Applications

The first priority in the comatose trauma patient is airway management. The performance of endotracheal intubation or cricothyrotomy during the early time period after injury may improve outcomes by protecting the patient from aspirating blood, vomitus, and secretions, and by permitting hyperventilation to decrease intracranial pressure. Use of the Glasgow coma scale—a clinical scale that assesses the depth and duration of impaired consciousness and coma by measuring motor responsiveness, verbal responsiveness, and eye opening—can produce consistency in observations of patients' levels of consciousness across observers and time.

This sentinel event indicator identifies an undesirable process of trauma patient care in which all occurrences warrant investigation.

Underlying factors that may influence indicator occurrences for this indicator are non-patient based. Identification, investigation, and analysis of one or more of these factors may assist in the interpretation of an organization's indicator data.

Examples of relevant non-patient based factors include:

1. adequacy of training and/or experience of physicians;

Source: Joint Commission on Accreditation of Healthcare Organizations: *IMSystem Indicators*. Oakbrook Terrace, IL: JCAHO, 1994, pp 187–193.

This indicator information set was developed to interpret data collected for IMSystem Indicator 22, which focuses on airway management of comatose trauma patients: *Comatose trauma patients with selected intracranial injuries discharged from the emergency department prior to endotracheal intubation or cricothyrotomy.*

FIGURE 3 (Continued)

2. adequacy of staffing of emergency department with physician(s);
3. adequacy of ongoing measurement, assessment, and improvement of physician performance;
4. adequacy of ongoing monitoring of patient's neurologic status by nursing personnel;
5. adequacy of staffing of emergency department with nursing personnel;
6. adequacy of ongoing measurement, assessment, and improvement of nursing personnel performance;
7. adequacy of supplies; and
8. equipment function status.

Terminology

Comatose

A Glasgow coma scale (GCS) score of less than or equal to 8 upon emergency department arrival.

Cricothyrotomy

An incision through the skin and cricothyroid membrane in the front of the neck to secure a patent (open) airway.

Emergency Department

The component of a health care organization that provides emergency services 24 hours per day, 365 days per year.

Emergency services are tasks performed by health professionals to benefit patients after the onset of a medical condition that manifests itself by symptoms of sufficient severity, including severe pain, that the lack of immediate medical attention could reasonably be expected by a prudent layperson who possesses an average knowledge of health and medicine to seriously jeopardize the patient's health, including danger of serious impairment to bodily functions or serious dysfunction of any bodily organ or part.

Emergency Department Arrival Date

The first recorded date that the patient had contact with the emergency department.

Continued on next page

FIGURE 3 Indicator Information Set for IMSystem Indicator 22 (Continued)

Emergency Department Arrival Time
The first recorded time (military time) that the patient had contact with the emergency department.

Emergency Department Disposition
Patient's location following discharge from the emergency department.

Endotracheal Intubation
The process of inserting an endotracheal tube into a patient's trachea (windpipe). An endotracheal tube is a hollow device used to administer anesthesia, maintain a patent (open) airway, ventilate the lungs, and/or prevent entrance of foreign material, such as stomach contents, into the tracheobronchial tree of the lungs. An endotracheal tube may be passed through a patient's mouth or nose, depending on clinical circumstances. An endotracheal tube is *not the same* as an oropharyngeal (or nasopharyngeal) tube (or airway), which is a hollow device extending from the mouth (or nose) to the pharynx (throat) but *not* entering the larynx (voicebox).

Glasgow Coma Scale (GCS) Score at Arrival
The first recorded GCS score within 15 minutes of emergency department arrival date and time (military time).

Intracranial Injuries
Identified by the presence of an ICD-9-CM[1] code for "Intracranial Injuries."

Location of Initial Care
Place of initial care for the patient.

Trauma Patients
Patients with an ICD-9-CM diagnosis code for "General Trauma Population" who are assessed in the ED and are then admitted to the hospital, transferred to another acute care hospital, or die in the emergency department.

[1]International Classification of Diseases, Ninth Revision, Clinical Modification

FIGURE 3 (Continued)

Note: *Also included are patients assessed in a trauma unit who have an ICD-9-CM diagnosis code for defining "General Trauma Population."*
Excluding:

- Patients whose *sole* trauma code is an isolated burn(s) as defined by ICD-9-CM diagnosis codes 940.0 to 949.5; or
- Patients 65 years of age or older whose *sole* trauma code is an isolated hip fracture, as defined by ICD-9-CM codes for "Hip Fractures."

Trauma Unit
The component of a health care organization that provides emergency *and* specialized intensive care to critically ill and injured patients.

Type of Airway Present at Emergency Department Disposition
The type of airway (endotracheal intubation or cricothyrotomy) used to control and maintain a patient's airway at ED disposition.

Data Collection Information

Population
Any patient for whom services were provided in the emergency department, a patient record was created, and the following criteria have been met:
Comatose trauma patients (defined as having a Glasgow coma scale score of 8 or less) with selected intracranial injuries defined by the presence of an ICD-9-CM code for "Intracranial Injuries" who are assessed in the emergency department and are then admitted to the hospital, are transferred to another acute care hospital, or die in the emergency department.

Exclusions
- See "Trauma Patients" exclusions; or
- Patients admitted directly to a trauma unit defined by *location of initial care* equal to "2" (see values for data elements on page 26-27).

Continued on next page

FIGURE 3 Indicator Information Set for IMSystem Indicator 22 (Continued)

Data Collection Approach

Retrospective—100%

Note: *Some hospitals may prefer to collect data concurrently by identifying patients in the population of interest as they enter the emergency department. It is important to note, however, that determining whether a patient meets criteria for inclusion in the trauma population rests in part on ICD-9-CM codes, which are typically assigned after patient discharge. Complete documentation and inclusion, therefore, of all relevant codes will require retrospective data collection.*

Data Accuracy

Indicator testing revealed variations and inaccuracies in Glasgow coma scale score documentation. The following guidelines should be followed when abstracting for the presence of GCS score:

- The *Glasgow* coma scale score is required rather than another type of trauma score. GCS score is composed of three components: eye opening response, best verbal response, and best motor response. The components are scored and then added together. The score must be a total of these three components and will range from 3 to 15. **Note:** *The actual number is required for arrival score only. Hourly measurements require a "yes/no" or "U" response.)*
- The arrival Glasgow coma scale score is taken *upon arrival* to the emergency department. Scores from ambulance run sheets are *not* acceptable as they were taken in route or outside of the emergency department patient care area.

Required Data Elements and Allowable Values

Emergency department arrival date   _ _/_ _/_ _ _ _
                               M M   D D   Y Y Y Y

Emergency department disposition   ___

1 = admitted to unmonitored bed

2 = admitted to telemetry (monitored bed)

3 = admitted to intensive care unit

4 = admitted to operating room

FIGURE 3 (Continued)

5 = transferred to another acute care facility
6 = discharged home
7 = left against medical advice
8 = expired

Glasgow Coma Scale (GCS) score at arrival   ___ ___
   3–15
99 = unknown/not documented

ICD-9-CM principal and other
   diagnosis codes   ___ ___ ___ . ___ ___

Location of initial care   ___
1 = emergency department
2 = trauma unit
99 = all other (includes inpatient units other than trauma units)

Type of airway present on emergency   ___
   department disposition
1 = endotracheal tube
2 = cricothyrotomy
3 = none

General Steps to Establish the Primary Indicator Rate
Primary Denominator
1. Identify patients with ICD-9-CM trauma codes for "Intracranial Injuries."
2. From #1, include only those patients with *location of initial care* equal to "1" and an *emergency department disposition* equal to "1–5" or "8."
3. Identify from #2 all patients who had a *Glasgow coma scale score at arrival* less than or equal to "8."

Primary Numerator
4. From #3, identify patients with *type of airway* equal to "3," or "none."
5. $\dfrac{\#4}{\#3} \times 100$ = primary indicator rate.

Continued on next page

FIGURE 3 Indicator Information Set for IMSystem Indicator 22 (Continued)

Indicator 22: Comotose trauma patients with selected intracranial injuries discharged from the Emergency Department (ED) prior to endotracheal intubation or cricothyrotomy

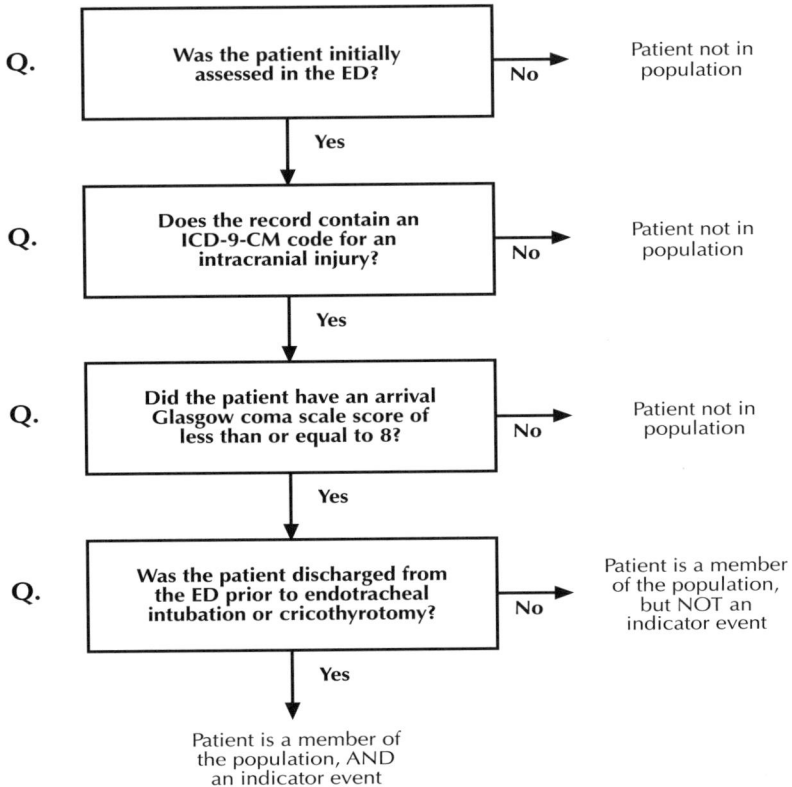

Q. **Was the patient initially assessed in the ED?** → No → Patient not in population

↓ Yes

Q. **Does the record contain an ICD-9-CM code for an intracranial injury?** → No → Patient not in population

↓ Yes

Q. **Did the patient have an arrival Glasgow coma scale score of less than or equal to 8?** → No → Patient not in population

↓ Yes

Q. **Was the patient discharged from the ED prior to endotracheal intubation or cricothyrotomy?** → No → Patient is a member of the population, but NOT an indicator event

↓ Yes

Patient is a member of the population, AND an indicator event

Simplified version of flow only, not intended for programming use (see *IMSystem Specifications Manual* for programmming algorithms).

Selected References

1. Gildenburg DL, Mabela M: Effect of early intubation and ventilation on outcome following head injury. In Dacey RG (ed): *Trauma of the Nervous System*. New York: Raven, 1985, pp 79–90.

2. Hemmer M: Ventilatory support for pulmonary failure of the head trauma patient. *Bull Eur Physiopathol Respir* 21:287–293, 1985.

3. Joint Commission on Accreditation of Healthcare Organizations: *Lexikon: Dictionary of Health Care Terms, Organizations, and Acronyms for the Era of Reform*. Oakbrook Terrace, IL: JCAHO, 1994.

4. Teasdale G, Jennett B: Assessment of coma and impaired consciousness: A practical scale. *Lancet* II:81–84, 1974.

TABLE 2 Six-Step Guide to Clinical Performance Data Interpretation

1. Select specific interpretation focus

2. Study characteristics of clinical performance data

3. Evaluate the strength of the data

4. Summarize the data

5. Study variation to identify undesirable variation

6. Determine underlying causes of undesirable variation

Sixth Interpretive Task: Determine Underlying Causes of Undesirable Variation

Interpreters who have diagnosed undesirable variation must direct their attention to identifying the underlying causes of the variation. This can be accomplished through various techniques. The approach described in Chapter Eight of this book involves constructing a flowchart, then a cause-and-effect diagram, followed by a Pareto diagram. A Pareto diagram is a special form of vertical bar graph that displays information in such a way that priorities for process improvement can be easily established. Brainstorming is a technique that is useful in generating the potential causes of variation for the cause-and-effect diagram. Because the number of potential causes may be very large, Pareto analysis enables interpreters to determine what causes are most important so that resources and attention are directed to areas where they will do the most good. Checksheets are a useful adjunct to Pareto analysis.

Summary Observations

The process of interpreting clinical performance data is divided into six ordered tasks (see Table 2, above). One or two points summarize the essence of each task.

1. *Selecting a specific data focus:* Interpreters must demonstrate restraint by selecting for interpretation a relatively modest amount of

FIGURE 4 Example of Control Chart for Beta Indicator ON-2

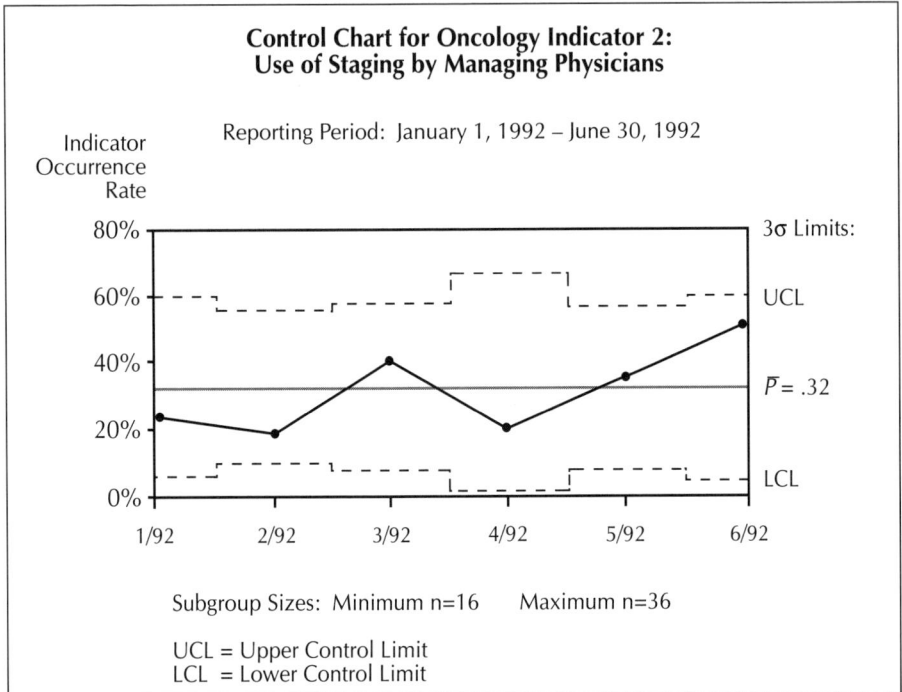

Control Chart for Oncology Indicator 2:
Use of Staging by Managing Physicians

Indicator Occurrence Rate

Reporting Period: January 1, 1992 – June 30, 1992

3σ Limits:

80%

60% — UCL

40%

$\overline{P} = .32$

20%

0% — LCL

1/92   2/92   3/92   4/92   5/92   6/92

Subgroup Sizes: Minimum n=16   Maximum n=36

UCL = Upper Control Limit
LCL = Lower Control Limit

The Joint Commission Oncology Care Task Force for Indicator Development developed the following ON-2 indicator for beta testing: *Patients undergoing treatment for primary cancer of the lung, colon/rectum, or female breast with American Joint Committee on Cancer (AJCC) stage of tumor designated by a managing physician.*

focused data. A useful unit of data for interpretation is an *indicator data set,* which is a collection of data generated by a common indicator.

   2. *Studying the characteristics of clinical performance data:* Data are devoid of meaning until interpreters learn what the data are measuring from the context in which the data arose. The *indicator information set* corresponding to an indicator data set provides that context. It also provides (or should provide) information about the important characteristics of the data.

   3. *Evaluating the strength of the data:* Interpreters must determine the strength of the data because this directly affects the strength of

FIGURE 5 Example of Comparison Chart for Beta Indicator ON-2

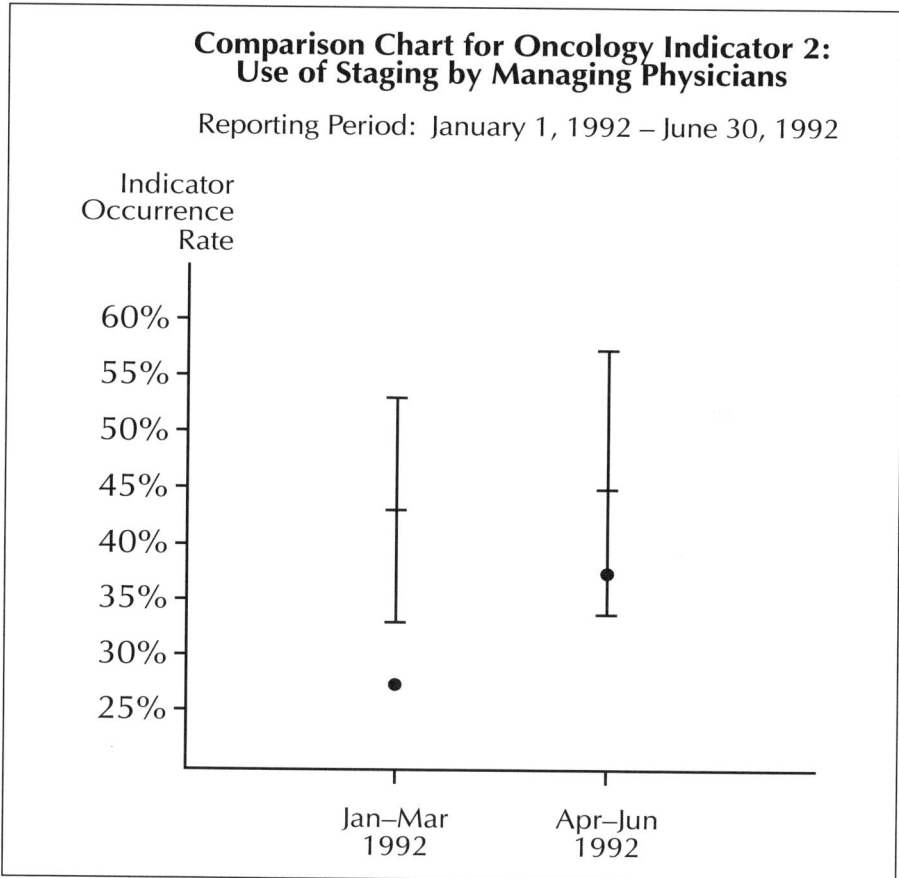

Comparison Chart for Oncology Indicator 2: Use of Staging by Managing Physicians

Reporting Period: January 1, 1992 – June 30, 1992

Indicator
Occurrence
Rate

60% –
55% –
50% –
45% –
40% –
35% –
30% –
25% –

Jan–Mar
1992

Apr–Jun
1992

The Joint Commission Oncology Care Task Force for Indicator Development developed the following ON-2 indicator for beta testing: *Patients undergoing treatment for primary cancer of the lung, colon/rectum, or female breast with American Joint Committee on Cancer (AJCC) stage of tumor designated by a managing physician.*

conclusions drawn from the data. If performance data cannot be trusted, neither can the performance information generated from them.

4. *Summarizing the data:* Raw data must be expressed in a frequency distribution that permits conclusions to be drawn, either directly or through further calculations, about the relationship between one series of observations and another.

5. *Studying variation to identify undesirable variation:* Variation is fluctuation in a series of results. A certain amount of variation is the inevitable product (output) of any system or process. Unusual, undesirable variation, however, can consume organization time and resources and may not contribute to the creation of value. Tools and techniques that aid in studying variation are the control chart and the comparison chart.

6. *Determining underlying causes of undesirable variation:* Flowcharts, cause-and-effect diagrams, and brainstorming are important tools and techniques that help interpreters identify underlying causes of variation. Pareto diagrams and checksheets help interpreters identify the "vital few" causes on which an organization's resources are best spent.

References

1.   Provost L, Leddick S: How to take multiple measures to get a complete picture of organizational performance. *National Productivity Review* pp 477–490, Autumn 1993.

2.   Joint Commission on Accreditation of Healthcare Organizations: *Primer on Indicator Development and Application.* Oakbrook Terrace, IL: JCAHO, 1990, pp 14–20.

3.   Bradford Hill, A: *Principles of Medical Statistics* 9th ed. New York: Oxford University Press, 1971, pp 51–69.

4.   Bounds G, Yorks L, Adams M, Ranney G. *Beyond Total Quality Management: Toward the Emerging Paradigm.* New York: McGraw-Hill, 1994, p 345.

5.   Walton M: *The Deming Management Method.* New York: Putnam Publishing Group, 1986, p 96.

6.   Shewhart WA: *Economic Control of Quality of Manufactured Product.* New York: Van Nostrand, 1931.

7.   Shewhart WA: *Statistical Method from the Viewpoint of Quality Control.* New York: Dover, 1986.

CHAPTER THREE

Selecting a Specific Interpretation Focus

Successful translation of clinical performance data into performance information requires selecting a data set that is sharply focused on a discrete clinical performance issue. One approach to locating such a data set is to focus on an *indicator data set.* An indicator data set is a collection of data generated by a single indicator that was developed to frame and quantify one or more important dimensions of a particular performance issue.

Examples of Indicator Data Sets

Three indicator data sets are depicted in Table 3 (see page 36). Each example reflects the summarized results of applying a single Joint Commission indicator (cardiovascular, oncology, or trauma) in several hundred hospitals during the beta phase of indicator development and testing. This testing process is described in detail elsewhere.[1]

Each column in Table 3 corresponds to a single indicator.

The data in the column labeled CV-7 belong to the cardiovascular care beta indicator:

> *Patients admitted for acute myocardial infarction (AMI),*
> *rule-out AMI, or unstable angina who have a discharge*

diagnosis of AMI, subcategorized by admission to an intensive care unit, a monitored bed, or an unmonitored bed.[*]

The data in the column labeled ON-7 belong to the oncology care beta indicator:

Patients undergoing pulmonary resection for primary lung cancer with postoperative complications of empyema, bronchopleural fistula, reoperation for postoperative bleeding, mechanical ventilation greater than five days postoperatively, or intrahospital death.[†]

The data in the column labeled TR-9 belong to the trauma care beta indicator:

Trauma patients transferred from initial receiving hospital to another acute care facility within six hours from emergency department (ED) arrival to ED departure.[‡]

A complete list of cardiovascular, oncology, and trauma care beta indicators is located in Appendix A.

---

[*] This indicator was developed by the Joint Commission Cardiovascular Care Task Force for Indicator Development between 1989 and 1991, and tested in numerous voluntary accredited hospitals between early 1992 and late 1993. It was recommended by the Cardiovascular Care Task Force and the Standards and Survey Procedures Committee, and approved by the Board of Commissioners for inclusion in the Joint Commission IMSystem pool of indicators. The final IMSystem form of the indicator is: *Patients admitted for acute myocardial infarction (AMI), rule-out AMI, or unstable angina who have a discharge diagnosis of AMI.*

[†] This indicator was developed by the Joint Commission Oncology Care Task Force for Indicator Development between 1989 and 1991, and tested in numerous voluntary accredited hospitals between early 1992 and late 1993. It was not recommended by the Oncology Care Task Force for inclusion in the Joint Commission IMSystem pool of indicators.

[‡] This indicator was developed by the Joint Commission Trauma Care Task Force for Indicator Development between 1989 and 1991, and tested in numerous voluntary accredited hospitals between early 1992 and late 1993. It was not recommended by the Trauma Care Task Force for inclusion in the Joint Commission IMSystem pool of indicators.

Readers who are unfamiliar with these indicator data sets might agree that the amount of data and information presented in Table 3 is relatively large and seemingly complex; yet this amount of data and information is not unusual for organizations' internal databases or data suppliers' external databases. Interpreters should not be intimidated by the numerous categories and the numbers in each category, but instead methodically select an indicator data set of interest, such as CV-7 or TR-9, and begin the interpretation process for that indicator data set.

Usefulness of Indicator Data Sets in Interpreting Clinical Performance Data

Indicator data sets are useful as focuses for interpreting clinical performance data for many reasons. *First, an indicator data set draws attention to the critical link between an indicator and the data it generates.* An indicator is developed, ideally by a group of clinical experts with the help of methodology experts, to frame important performance issues and then quantify performance related to those issues. An indicator queries an organization about an important patient care process or health care outcome; the data set then generated provides the basic material to address the query. *An indicator provides the frame of reference, or context, for assigning meaning to all relevant indicator data.*

Consider, for example, the Joint Commission IMSystem indicator that focuses on diagnostic accuracy for patients with congestive heart failure:

> *Patients with principal discharge diagnosis of congestive heart failure having documented etiology.**

---

* This indicator was developed by the Joint Commission Cardiovascular Care Task Force for Indicator Development between 1989 and 1991, and tested in numerous voluntary accredited hospitals between early 1992 and late 1993. It was recommended by the Cardiovascular Task Force and the Standards and Survey Procedures Committee and approved by the Board of Commissioners for inclusion in the Joint Commission IMSystem pool of indicators.

TABLE 3 Joint Commission Beta Testing Data Sets for Selected Cardiovascular, Oncology, and Trauma Care Indicators

Total Database Description	CV-7	ON-7	TR-9
I: Insufficient information to determine denominator status	9,510	7,578	0
II: Not part of the indicator population	94,921	53,051	67,748
III: Insufficient information to determine numerator status	0	66	57
IV: Indicator denominator, but not numerator	60,296	2,725	57
V: Indicator numerator, but not denominator	44,808	719	1,510
Overall indicator rate = V ÷ (IV+V)	42.6	20.9	96.4
Percent of trauma population not eligible for indicator population = II ÷ (I+II+III+IV+V)	45.3	82.7	97.7
Percent of potential numerator or denominator cases lost due to missing data = (I+III) ÷ (I+III+IV+V)	8.3	68.9	3.5
Hospital Level Description			
Number of hospitals reporting denominator cases for this indicator	192	164	80
Median hospital indicator rate	46.4	20	100
Interquartile range indicator rate	(30.2, 74.2)	(7.6, 33.3)	(97.0, 100)
Median hospital denominator cases	354	13	8
Interquartile range for denominator cases	(144, 755)	(5, 28)	(3, 25)
Median hospital percent not eligible	42.5	24.4	92.3
Interquartile range for percent not eligible	(31.4, 58.4)	(2.5, 74.1)	(82.7, 98.6)
Median hospital percent missing	1.5	89.8	0
Interquartile range for percent missing	(0, 7.3)	(83.1, 94.0)	(0, 0)

Source: Joint Commission beta database

The performance issue here is how well clinicians diagnose and document etiology of congestive heart failure (CHF) for patients with this syndrome. Effective and appropriate treatment of CHF depends on understanding the cause of the underlying heart disease. The treatment for the patient with CHF caused by hypertension, for example, is quite different from the treatment for the patient with CHF caused by hyperthyroidism or valvular heart disease. The inability of clinicians to distinguish among causes or consider the issue of causation can result in undesirable patient health outcomes, including preventable death.

Indicator-driven performance data provide the material for determining how well an organization and its clinicians are performing in this important process of care. The indicator provides the frame of reference for best interpreting the indicator data. From the perspective of an individual hospital, for example, a data set for the CHF indicator might include measurements for 220 patients who carry a diagnosis of CHF, only 80 of whom have the etiology for their CHF documented in the patient record. The hospital's indicator rate of approximately 36% would alert informed data users (those who understand the frame of reference for assigning meaning to the data) to the need for improvement in this clinical area. Most clinicians would agree that the number of patients with documented etiology of CHF in their records should approach 100%.

How important to interpreting data accurately is an understanding of the link between a clinical performance data set and its parent indicator? Health care providers who do not have an understanding of the context in which data are produced can seriously misinterpret the data.

Consider, for example, the Joint Commission IMSystem indicator that focuses on the ongoing monitoring of trauma patients in the emergency department:

> *Trauma patients with blood pressure, pulse, and respiration documented on arrival and hourly for three hours,*

or until emergency department disposition, whichever is earlier.*

This indicator measures how well organizations monitor seriously injured and potentially seriously injured patients—that is, patients with *International Classification of Diseases, Ninth Revision, Clinical Modification* (ICD-9-CM) trauma diagnoses who are admitted to the operating room or intensive care unit of the hospital, who die in the emergency department, or who are transferred to another acute care facility. This indicator *does not measure* the ongoing monitoring ability of organizations for injured but stable patients who are discharged to home or admitted to an unmonitored hospital bed.

Consider a clinician interpreter who is only superficially acquainted or not acquainted at all with the trauma indicator that produced a rate of 9.7% for his or her hospital. Despite a lack of knowledge about the context of the data, the individual may judge the rate acceptable because it has been erroneously assumed that the population monitored by the indicator includes patients with all kinds of traumatic injuries, however minor. Hourly vital signs, the clinician may reason, would be inappropriate for the vast majority of "trauma" patients (for example, patients with scrapes, bruises, simple lacerations, or simple fractures), thus resulting in a relatively low indicator rate of 9.7%. The clinician may even express annoyance at what he or she perceives as an externally imposed, inappropriate requirement to monitor hourly vital signs on all "trauma" patients, however slight their injuries, especially in a busy emergency setting where staff may already be overextended in meeting the needs of patients.

---

* This indicator was developed by the Joint Commission Trauma Care Task Force for Indicator Development between 1989 and 1991, and tested in numerous voluntary accredited hospitals between early 1992 and late 1993. It was recommended by the Trauma Care Task Force and the Standards and Survey Procedures Committee and approved by the Board of Commissioners for inclusion in the Joint Commission IMSystem pool of indicators.

For clinician interpreters who understand the indicator's true frame of reference, a rate of 9.7% is cause for concern. The indicator rate should approach 100%, meaning that most patients destined for the operating room, intensive care unit, morgue, or transfer to another acute care facility should receive *at least* hourly vital signs as part of their care in the emergency department. Most people would agree that this is a realistic expectation. The clinician described in the previous paragraph who understands the correct frame of reference in which to interpret the data would likely agree with this assessment of the 9.7% rate. He or she would also likely mobilize resources rapidly to diagnose and remedy the underlying sources of the undesirable variation observed between actual (9.7%) and desired (approaching 100%) practice.

Second, indicator data sets set the stage for learning all the characteristics of the performance data defined by the set. Study of these characteristics forms the second task of a formal approach to clinical performance data interpretation and is the subject of Chapter Four.

Third, indicator data sets yield an abundance of performance data and information in addition to simple indicator rates. Studying an indicator's *algorithm*, the sequence of steps, is the most direct route to obtaining this additional data and information. An indicator's algorithm is developed and used to classify data elements and to calculate all indicator data measurements.

For instance, consider the Joint Commission's algorithm (see Figure 6, page 40) for the trauma care beta indicator that measures the efficiency of prehospital emergency medical services:

*Trauma patients with prehospital emergency medical services scene time greater than 20 minutes.**

---

* This indicator was developed by the Joint Commission Trauma Care Task Force for Indicator Development between 1989 and 1991, and tested in numerous voluntary accredited hospitals between early 1992 and late 1993. It was recommended by the Trauma Care Task Force and the Standards and Survey Procedures Committee and approved by the Board of Commissioners for inclusion in the Joint Commission IMSystem pool of indicators.

FIGURE 6 Joint Commission TR-1 Indicator Algorithm

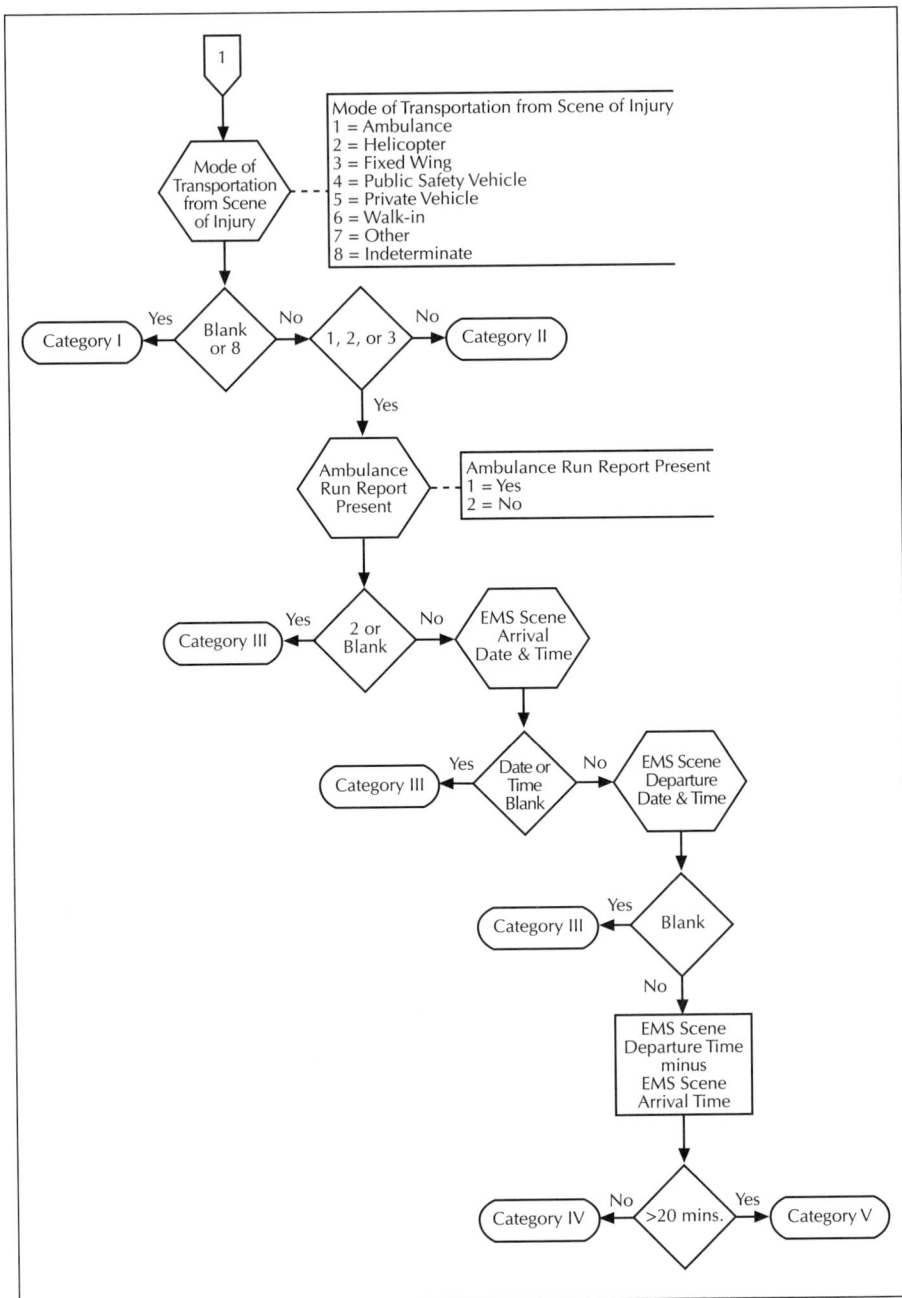

This algorithm corresponds to the beta indicator: *Trauma patients with prehospital emergency medical services scene times of greater than 20 minutes.*

The rationale behind this indicator is that time spent in the prehospital phase of care may be related to outcomes of morbidity and mortality because the condition of critically injured patients frequently deteriorates over time. Thus, except for problems in patient extrication, trauma patients should be transported with minimal delay.

The overall indicator rate for the 158 hospitals that submitted data to the Joint Commission's beta phase database during 1992 to 1993 was 25.3%, meaning that scene times were greater than 20 minutes in 25.3% of cases. While this measurement directly answers the question posed by the indicator, there are other questions indirectly posed by the indicator that are answered as well.

Further analysis of the algorithm, for instance, reveals the number of trauma patients for whom an emergency medical services run report is present in the patient record. These data are important because hospitals in which ambulance run reports are missing in patient records, say 90% of the time, first need to improve this process of care (that is, include run reports in patient records) before they can even begin to assess level of performance relative to length of prehospital scene times.

Fourth, when indicator data sets are missing or otherwise unavailable, interpreters are duly forewarned that data dredging will be required to interpret the data. Data dredging (also called *data mining*) is the process of developing indicators after, rather than before, data are collected. This approach enjoys some popularity. It is used, for instance, each time data elements for performance improvement activities are drawn from a third-party payer claims database. It is used each time registries' numerous variables are used for research purposes. Perusing the data elements in claims databases or registries is sometimes useful in identifying possible indicators. However, as described below, this approach to indicator development may be less efficient than framing performance issues first with indicators and then collecting data that address the issue.

Indicator development, according to many experts, is a discrete process that requires adequate time and resources to produce a reliable and valid product.[1] Developing indicators by data dredging an existing claims database or registry has several drawbacks:

- It adds considerable work to interpreting data, which is frequently a challenging endeavor, especially to health professionals inexperienced in the process.
- It restricts indicator developers to using data elements available in the claims database or registry. These data elements may not meet their needs in developing meaningful indicators and addressing important performance issues.
- It raises serious questions about the reliability and validity of indicators developed after data collection, which are subject to the same requirements of data strength as indicators developed before data collection.

Finally, indicator data sets provide a structured means to conceptualizing data, which can result in more efficient use of resources and increased production of valid and reliable performance information. The sheer amount of indicator data requiring interpretation can be overwhelming, especially when a clear method for approaching the data is unknown or not applied. Discrete indicator data sets are convenient and meaningful "packages" for performing interpretive tasks.

When interpreters lack familiarity with indicator data sets, they also probably lack familiarity with indicators and the clinical performance issues they frame and quantify. Without the necessary knowledge base, these interpreters must struggle along in the interpretive process, falsely guided by numbers alone, rather than by the issues and inquiries to which the numbers should guide them. This can lead to a distorted regard for data and information that bear no relationship to reality whatsoever. In these circumstances, information derived from performance measurement activities will not likely meet the decision-making needs of potential information users. A much more efficient and meaningful approach to interpreting data is achieved by understanding of indicators and indicator measurement systems.

Limitation of Individual Indicator Data Sets

The simplicity of indicator data sets enhances their appeal as a focus for data interpretation. They possess, however, one major limitation: they typically provide information about only one dimension of a clinical performance issue. This amount of information would be inadequate when information about multiple dimensions is needed to fully assess a performance issue. Organizations, for example, may focus their efforts on improving a discrete dimension of performance (such as timeliness of a service), but if they do so at the expense of another dimension (such as patient safety), the aim of improving performance has been defeated.

Interpreters must be prepared to expand their data focus to include a *family of indicator data sets*, in which each set reflects a different dimension of performance related to the same clinical performance issue. In this way, a full picture of performance can be obtained.[2]

Consider, for instance, the Joint Commission IMSystem indicator that measures extended postoperative stays in patients undergoing coronary artery bypass graft procedures:

> *Patients undergoing isolated coronary artery bypass graft procedures: number of days from surgery to discharge.**

Whether the right operation was performed (dimension of appropriateness) and was performed in the correct manner (dimension of

---

* The following indicator was developed by the Joint Commission Cardiovascular Care Task Force for Indicator Development between 1989 and 1991, and tested in numerous voluntary accredited hospitals between early 1992 and late 1993: *Patients with prolonged postoperative stay for isolated coronary artery bypass graft (CABG) procedures, subcategorized by initial or subsequent CABG procedures, by emergent or nonemergent procedures, and by the use or nonuse of a circulatory support device.* It was recommended by the Cardiovascular Care Task Force and the Standards and Survey Procedures Committee and approved by the Board of Commissioners for inclusion in the Joint Commission IMSystem pool of indicators.

effectiveness) are as important to patients as how the number of days they spend in the hospital compares to the average.

Or consider the Joint Commission IMSystem indicator that measures diagnostic accuracy and resource utilization for patients admitted for acute myocardial infarction (AMI), rule-out AMI, or unstable angina:

> *Patients admitted for acute myocardial infarction (AMI), rule-out AMI, or unstable angina who have a discharge diagnosis of AMI.*[*]

For patients with chest pain or related ischemic symptoms that are consistent with AMI, whether or not clinicians accurately diagnose their condition, is as important as the hospital's efficient use of resources over time.

Finally, consider the Joint Commission IMSystem indicator that measures the availability of data for diagnosing and staging major types of cancer:

> *Patients undergoing resections for primary cancer of the female breast, lung, or colon/rectum for whom a surgical pathology consultation report (pathology report) is present in the patient record.*[†]

---

[*] This indicator was developed by the Joint Commission Cardiovascular Care Task Force for Indicator Development between 1989 and 1991, and tested in numerous voluntary accredited hospitals between early 1992 and late 1993. It was recommended by the Cardiovascular Care Task Force and the Standards and Survey Procedures Committee, and approved by the Board of Commissioners for inclusion in the Joint Commission IMSystem pool of indicators. The final IMSystem form of the indicator is: *Patients admitted for acute myocardial infarction (AMI), rule-out AMI, or unstable angina who have a discharge diagnosis of AMI.*

[†] This indicator was developed by the Joint Commission Oncology Care Task Force for Indicator Development between 1989 and 1991, and tested in numerous voluntary accredited hospitals between early 1992 and late 1993. It was recommended by the Oncology Care Task Force and the Standards and Survey Procedures Committee and approved by the Board of Commissioners for inclusion in the Joint Commission IMSystem pool of indicators.

Whether clinicians correctly diagnose and stage the cancer based on surgical pathology reports is as important to cancer patients as the presence of pathology reports in their records.

Summary Observations

Health care providers must be realistic about their ability to manage and interpret clinical performance data. There are several important observations to be gleaned from this chapter about the first task of a formal approach to interpretation.

1. The ability to effectively interpret clinical performance data depends on the ability to sharply focus on a discrete clinical performance issue and sustain that focus throughout the interpretation process. An indicator data set provides a logical and useful interpretation focus.

2. An indicator data set is a collection of data generated by applying an indicator that frames and quantifies one or more important dimensions of a performance issue.

3. An indicator data set is useful as a focus for data interpretation because:

- It draws attention to the critical link between an indicator and the data it generates.
- It sets the stage for learning all the characteristics of the performance data defined by the set.
- It yields an abundance of performance data and information in addition to simple indicator rates.
- When it is missing or otherwise unavailable, interpreters are forewarned that data dredging will be required to interpret the data.
- It provides a structured means to conceptualizing data, which can result in more efficient use of resources and increased production of valid and reliable performance information.

4. One limitation of an indicator data set is that it typically focuses on a discrete dimension of performance related to a clinical performance issue. Interpreters must be prepared to expand their data focus to include a family of indicator data sets in which each set reflects a different dimension of performance related to the same clinical performance issue. In this way a full picture of performance can be obtained.

References

1.   Joint Commission on Accreditation of Healthcare Organizations: *Primer on Indicator Development and Application.* Oakbrook Terrace, IL: JCAHO, 1990.

2.   Provost L, Leddick S: How to take multiple measures to get a complete picture of organizational performance. *National Productivity Review* pp 477–490, Autumn 1993.

CHAPTER FOUR

Studying Characteristics of Clinical Performance Data

M any interpreters encountering clinical performance data for the first time are surprised that the meaning of the data is not self-evident. Consider, for instance, a hospital's 66-minute average time to assess and move patients with specified injuries or illnesses from the emergency department to the operating room for surgery. The exact meaning of this piece of data (66-minute average time) is not apparent to many people. Or, for example, a hospital discharges 11 comatose patients from its emergency department to in-hospital destinations. Nine patients are endotracheally intubated, one has a cricothyrotomy, and one has no mechanical airway in place. The precise meaning of these data (nine comatose patients with intubations, one with a cricothyrotomy, and one with neither procedure) may similarly elude many people.

Making sense of clinical performance data requires knowing the context for the data. To find a description of this context requires studying the characteristics of the indicator that generated the data. As described in the previous chapter, an indicator provides the frame of reference for assigning meaning to all relevant data.

Studying important characteristics of clinical performance data answers five questions:

- Which dimension(s) of performance do the data measure?
- Do the data measure a patient care process or patient health care outcome?
- Do the data measure many events or phenomena or an individual event or phenomenon?
- Are the data reported as a continuous variable or discrete variable?
- Do the data measure a desirable or an undesirable outcome or process?

Dimensions of Performance Assessed by Clinical Performance Data

There are at least nine measurable dimensions of performance that may be assessed by clinical performance data. These dimensions include efficacy, appropriateness, availability, timeliness, effectiveness, continuity, safety, efficiency, and respect and caring (see Table 1, page 4).[1, 2] The importance of these performance dimensions lies both in their individual and their collective impact on patient health outcomes, costs, and judgments of quality and value.

Efficacy of a procedure or treatment in relation to a patient's condition is the degree to which the care or intervention has been shown to accomplish the desired or projected outcome(s) for patients.[1] Efficacy addresses how much the care actually benefits patients and, at a minimum, does no harm. Inefficacious treatments and procedures are virtually always inappropriate and waste health care resources.[2] Doing the right thing for patients requires the use of efficacious care or interventions.[1]

The appropriateness of a specific test, procedure, or service is the degree to which the care or intervention provided is relevant to a patient's clinical needs, given the current state of knowledge.[1] Appropriateness issues have probably received the most widespread attention among all the dimensions of performance because inappropriate tests, procedures, treatments, and services cost money and waste health care resources. The current obligation to reduce health care expenditures is not the only issue relating to appropriateness. Most procedures, services, treatments, and tests carry a measurable risk of complication to patients. Patients who do not need a particular test or service should not be subjected to its risks. Like efficacy, appropriateness entails doing the right thing for patients.[1]

Clinical performance data that quantify appropriateness are collected by measuring, for example, whether comatose trauma patients (Glasgow Coma Scale score equal to eight or less) have had their airways managed correctly before being discharged from the emergency department to other in-hospital destinations.* The first priority in the comatose patient is establishing a mechanical airway either by intubating the patient or performing a cricothyrotomy. Establishing a mechanical airway not only secures an unobstructed passageway to the lungs for ventilation but protects the patient from aspirating blood, vomitus, and secretions. It also permits hyperventilation to decrease intracranial pressure.

Another measure of appropriateness would be data showing whether patients undergoing resections for primary colorectal cancer have had their entire colon examined as part of their preoperative evaluation.† Relevant information, such as the existence of metastases, is gained by examining the entire colon. This information determines the need for further preoperative staging evaluation and guides planning for the extent of surgery. Examination of the entire colon is proof of the thoroughness of the preoperative evaluation and bears directly on care management and patient survival.

The availability of a needed test, procedure, treatment, or service to a patient is the degree to which appropriate care or intervention is

---

* These data are generated by applying the following Joint Commission IMSystem indicator: *Comatose trauma patients with selected intracranial injuries discharged from the emergency department prior to endotracheal intubation or cricothyrotomy.*

† These data are generated by applying the following IMSystem indicator: *Patients with resections of primary colorectal cancer whose preoperative evaluation, by a managing physician, includes examination of the entire colon.*

obtainable when required by a patient.[1] A health care service is available when it can be obtained from appropriate personnel at the time and place it is needed. The availability dimension of performance does not entail doing the right thing for patients as much as it involves doing the right thing *well,* as do the rest of the dimensions of performance.[1]

Availability can be measured by showing, for example, whether pathology reports containing important information for diagnosis and staging (such as histological type, invasion or extension, lymph node examination, and status of margins) are present in the medical records of patients undergoing resections for certain kinds of cancer.* Obtaining this information is critical for physicians to select appropriate and effective treatment plans. Unavailability of pathology reports, for whatever reason, can result in inappropriate or inadequate treatments.

The timeliness with which a test, procedure, treatment, or service provided to a patient is the degree to which the care or intervention is provided to the patient at the most beneficial or necessary time.[1] Timeliness can be measured by showing, for example, how quickly patients with specified injuries are assessed and moved from the emergency department to the operating room for needed surgical procedures.†

The effectiveness with which tests, procedures, treatments, and services are provided is the degree to which the care or intervention is provided in the correct manner, given the current state of knowledge, in order to achieve the desired or projected outcome for the patient.[1] Effectiveness can be assessed by showing, for example, the

---

* These data are generated by applying the following IMSystem indicator: *Patients undergoing resections for primary cancer of the female breast, lung, or colon/rectum for whom a surgical pathology consultation report (pathology report) is present in the medical record.*
† These data are generated by applying the following IMSystem indicator: *Trauma patients undergoing selected neurosurgical, orthopedic, or abdominal surgical procedures: time from emergency department arrival to induction of anesthesia.*

in-hospital mortality rate of cardiovascular patients undergoing percutaneous transluminal coronary angioplasty (PTCA).* Increased postoperative mortality for PTCA patients, in comparison to peer institutions, raises questions about effectiveness of care or intervention.

The continuity of the services provided to the patient with respect to other services, practitioners, and providers and over time is the degree to which the care or intervention for the patient is coordinated among practitioners, among organizations, and over time.[1] Continuity is quantified by showing, for example, the extent to which estrogen receptor diagnostic analysis results are present in the records of female patients with Stage II or greater primary breast cancer who are undergoing initial biopsy or resection.† Obtaining and communicating estrogen receptor diagnostic analysis results is important in diagnosing, estimating prognosis, and managing the care of female patients with breast cancer. When these test results are missing, coordination of patient care among practitioners, among organizations, and over time becomes difficult.

Safety is the degree to which the risk of an intervention and risk in the care environment are reduced for the patient and others, including the health care provider.[1] Safety can be measured by showing, for instance, the incidence of medication errors, blood transfusion reactions, or organization-specific mortality for certain procedures.

The efficiency with which services are provided is the relationship between the outcomes (results of care) and the resources used to deliver the care.[1] Efficiency can be assessed by showing, for

---

* These data are generated by applying the following IMSystem indicator: *Intrahospital mortality of cardiovascular patients undergoing isolated coronary artery bypass graft surgery, undergoing percutaneous transluminal angioplasty, or with a principal diagnosis of acute myocardial infarction.*

† These data are generated by applying the following IMSystem indicator: *Female patients with Stage II or greater primary breast cancer, undergoing initial biopsy or resection, who have estrogen receptor diagnostic analysis results in the medical record.*

example, the rate at which patients admitted with a diagnosis of AMI, rule-out AMI, or unstable angina are discharged from the hospital with a diagnosis of acute myocardial infarction (AMI).* Both underadmission and overadmission of these patients signal inefficiency. In the first case, the results of care may be quite poor (such as death) even though resources used to deliver the care were minimal over time (patients were not admitted to the hospital). In the second case, the results of care may be acceptable (patients did not have an AMI but spent one or two days in the hospital) but the amount of resources used was higher.

The respect and caring with which services are provided is the degree to which the patient or a designee is involved in care decisions and to which those providing services do so with sensitivity and respect for the patient's needs, expectations, and individual differences.[1] Data that measure respect and caring show how satisfied patients are with their health care providers.

Outcome Versus Process Clinical Performance Data

Clinical performance data are quantifications of either an outcome or a process of care. *Outcome data* are quantifications of a specified outcome. *Outcome* is defined here as the cumulative effect at a defined point in time of performing one or more processes in the care of a patient.[3] Patient survival and death are two examples of outcomes. Examples of clinical performance outcome data include the following:

- A health care network's rate of 45% for patients admitted for AMI, rule-out AMI, or unstable angina who have a discharge diagnosis of AMI;*
- An intrahospital mortality rate of 6% for cardiovascular patients

---

* These data are generated by applying the following IMSystem indicator: *Patients admitted for acute myocardial infarction (AMI), rule-out AMI, or unstable angina who have a discharge diagnosis of AMI.*

undergoing isolated coronary artery bypass graft surgery;* and

- An intrahospital mortality rate of 100% for trauma patients with a systolic blood pressure of less than 70 mm Hg within two hours of emergency department arrival who did not undergo a laparotomy or thoracotomy.†

Process data are quantifications of what is done to, for, or by patients, as in performance of an activity, a service, or a procedure. The best process data focus on processes that are closely linked to outcomes, meaning that a scientific basis exists for believing that the process, when executed well, will increase the probability of achieving a desired outcome. Examples of process data include the following:

- A hospital rate of 30% for oncology patients undergoing resections for primary cancer of the female breast, lung, or colon/rectum for whom a surgical pathology consultation report (pathology report) is present in the patient record.‡

- A hospital rate of 75% for oncology patients undergoing treatment for primary cancer of the female breast, lung, or colon/rectum having stage of tumor designated by a managing physician.§

---

* These data are generated by applying the following IMSystem indicator: *Intrahospital mortality of cardiovascular patients undergoing isolated coronary artery bypass graft surgery, undergoing percutaneous transluminal angioplasty, or with a principal diagnosis of acute myocardial infarction.*

† These data are generated by applying the following IMSystem indicator: *Intrahospital mortality or trauma patients with a systolic blood pressure of less than 70 mm Hg anytime within two hours of emergency department arrival who did not undergo a laparotomy or thoracotomy.*

‡ These data are generated by applying the following IMSystem indicator: *Patients undergoing resections for primary cancer of the female breast, lung, or colon/rectum for whom a surgical pathology consultation report (pathology report) is present in the medical record.*

§ These data are generated by applying the following IMSystem indicator: *Patients undergoing treatment for primary cancer of the female breast, lung, or colon/rectum having stage of tumor designated by a managing physician.*

Aggregate Versus Sentinel Event Clinical Performance Data

Clinical performance data may express information about many events or phenomena (aggregate performance data) or about an individual event or phenomenon (sentinel event data) (see Figure 7, page 55). *Sentinel event data* are quantifications of individual events that are usually rare, adverse, and frequently avoidable. Sentinel event data include:

- Comatose trauma patients with selected intracranial injuries discharged from the emergency department prior to endotracheal intubation or cricothyrotomy;* and
- Intrahospital mortality of trauma patients with a diagnosis of pneumothorax or hemothorax who did not undergo a thoracostomy or thoracotomy.[†]

Aggregate performance data are quantifications of many events or phenomena, a certain proportion of which are expected (even if they are undesirable). Aggregate performance data may be collected on, for example:

- Patients with Stage II or greater primary breast cancer, undergoing initial biopsy or resection, who have estrogen receptor diagnostic analysis results in the patient record.[‡]

Aggregate performance data, as described elsewhere, have several advantages over sentinel event performance data.[4] Briefly,

---

* These data are generated by applying the following Joint Commission IMSystem indicator: *Comatose trauma patients with selected intracranial injuries discharged from the emergency department prior to endotracheal intubation or cricothyrotomy.*

† These data are generated by applying the following IMSystem indicator: *Intrahospital mortality of trauma patients with a diagnosis of pneumothorax or hemothorax who did not undergo a thoracostomy or thoracotomy.*

‡ These data are generated by applying the following IMSystem indicator: *Female patients with Stage II or greater primary breast cancer, undergoing initial biopsy or resection, who have estrogen receptor diagnostic analysis results in the medical record.*

FIGURE 7 Indicator Relationships

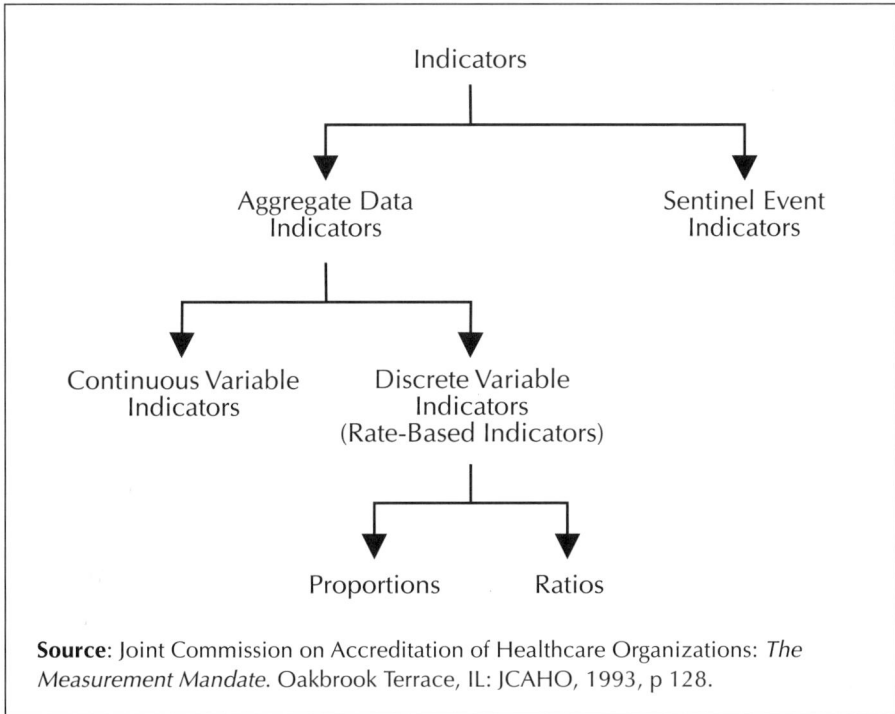

```
                        Indicators
                            |
         +------------------+------------------+
         |                                     |
   Aggregate Data                        Sentinel Event
     Indicators                            Indicators
         |
   +-----+-----------------+
   |                       |
Continuous Variable   Discrete Variable
   Indicators            Indicators
                    (Rate-Based Indicators)
                            |
                     +------+------+
                     |             |
                Proportions      Ratios
```

Source: Joint Commission on Accreditation of Healthcare Organizations: *The Measurement Mandate*. Oakbrook Terrace, IL: JCAHO, 1993, p 128.

This figure shows how the various types of indicators are related.

sentinel event data represent the extremes of performance measurement, and their most practical applications tend to relate to risk-management activities. Even then, analysis and investigation of a sentinel event may prove to be inconclusive. Aggregate performance data, by contrast, are notable for their ability to guide organizations in improving their norms of performance, rather than focusing exclusively on censoring or eliminating individual outliers.

Continuous Variable Versus Discrete Variable Clinical Performance Data

Aggregate performance data can be reported as either continuous variable data or discrete variable data. (Discrete variable data were previously called rate-based data.) (See Figure 7.) *Continuous variable data* are quantifications of events or phenomena that, when measured, have a potentially infinite number of possible values along a continuum. Continuous variable data are collected on, for example:

- Trauma patients undergoing selected neurosurgical, orthopedic, or abdominal surgical procedures: time from emergency department arrival to procedure;*
- Trauma patients with head computerized tomography (CT) scan performed: time from emergency department arrival to initial CT scan;†
- Patients undergoing isolated coronary artery bypass graft procedures: number of days from surgery to discharge;‡ and
- Patients undergoing percutaneous transluminal coronary angioplasty: number of days from procedure to discharge.§

In each of these examples, time is the continuum along which the events of interest are measured. There are an infinite number of time values—10 minutes, 60 minutes, 600 minutes—from emergency department arrival to performing a surgical procedure.

Discrete variable (attribute) data are quantifications of events or phenomena that, when measured, fall into one of at least two categories (for example, "yes or no" or "unknown"; less than 20 minutes or greater than 20 minutes). Discrete variable data are known widely in biostatistics as *attribute data*. Both terms are

---

* These data are generated by applying the following IMSystem indicator: *Trauma patients undergoing selected neurosurgical, orthopedic, or abdominal surgical procedures: time from emergency department arrival to induction of anesthesia.*

† These data are generated by applying the following IMSystem indicator: *Trauma patients with head computerized tomography (CT) scan performed: time from emergency department arrival to initial CT scan.*

‡ These data are generated by applying the following IMSystem indicator: *Patients undergoing isolated coronary artery bypass graft procedures: number of days from surgery to discharge.*

§ These data are generated by applying the following IMSystem indicator: *Patients undergoing percutaneous transluminal coronary angioplasty: number of days from procedure to discharge.*

entrenched in the literature and are used interchangeably throughout this book.

Discrete variable data are being collected in the following examples:

- Patients with a principal discharge diagnosis of congestive heart failure having documented etiology (the etiology is either documented or not documented);*
- Intrahospital mortality of cardiovascular patients undergoing isolated coronary artery bypass graft surgery, undergoing percutaneous transluminal angioplasty, or with a principal diagnosis of AMI (the patient either dies or does not die);†
- Patients with resections of primary colorectal cancer whose preoperative evaluation, by a managing physician, includes examination of the entire colon (the entire colon is either examined or it is not examined);‡
- Trauma patients with selected intracranial injuries with Glasgow Coma Scale score documented on arrival and hourly for three hours, or until emergency department disposition, whichever is earlier (the Glasgow Coma Scale score is either documented or it is not documented).§

The type of data—continuous versus attribute—undergoing

---

* These data are generated by applying the following IMSystem indicator: *Patients with principal discharge diagnosis of congestive heart failure having a documented etiology.*

† These data are generated by applying the following IMSystem indicator: *Intrahospital mortality of cardiovascular patients undergoing isolated coronary artery bypass graft surgery, undergoing percutaneous transluminal angioplasty, or with a principal diagnosis of acute myocardial infarction.*

‡ These data are generated by applying the following IMSystem indicator: *Patients with resections of primary colorectal cancer whose preoperative evaluation, by a managing physician, includes examination of the entire colon.*

§ These data are generated by applying the following IMSystem indicator: *Trauma patients with selected intracranial injuries with Glasgow Coma Scale score documented on arrival and at least hourly for three hours or until emergency department disposition, whichever is earlier.*

interpretation has broad implications for the type of control chart used to study variation (variables control chart versus attribute control chart; see Chapter Seven). The Joint Commission has had the most experience with attribute data because most of the beta indicators produced attribute data. Post-beta phase modifications of some attribute indicators resulted in continuous data indicators for the same performance issue. For example, consider the following beta indicator that produced attribute data:

> *Trauma patients with diagnosis of laceration of the liver or spleen, requiring surgery, undergoing laparotomy greater than two hours after emergency department arrival, subcategorized by pediatric or adult patients.**

This indicator was changed to a continuous data indicator, based on test data. The new indicator, now part of the IMSystem, reads as follows:

> *Trauma patients undergoing selected [neurological, orthopedic, or] abdominal surgical procedures: time from emergency department arrival to procedure.†*

The amount of information conveyed by continuous data is much greater than for attribute data. With continuous data, health care organizations can know with precision their average times from emergency department arrival to procedure for patients undergoing selected abdominal surgical procedures. With attribute data, organizations can know only how many surgical patients made or did not make the two-hour cutoff point.

Discrete variable data are also known as *categorical data*. Categorical data comprise two categories: nominal data and ordinal data.[5] *Nominal data* are qualitative data with categories that have no inherent

---

* This indicator was developed for the Joint Commission Trauma Care Task Force for Indicator Development.

† These data are generated by applying the following IMSystem indicator: *Trauma patients undergoing selected neurosurgical, orthopedic, or abdominal surgical procedures: time from emergency department arrival to induction of anesthesia.*

ranking. For instance, data listing marital status as single, married, divorced, or separated are nominal data. *Ordinal data* are qualitative data categories that are ranked, but there is no natural numerical distance between the possible values. Only the relative sizes of numbers are important. For instance, data describing symptoms as absent, mild, moderate, or severe are examples of ordinal data.

Desirable Versus Undesirable Clinical Performance Data

Clinical performance data are quantifications of processes or outcomes that are either desirable or undesirable. Examples of clinical performance data that quantify desirable processes or outcomes are:

- Trauma patients with blood pressure, pulse, and respiration documented on arrival and at least hourly for three hours or until emergency department disposition, whichever is earlier (documentation of hourly vital signs is a desirable process of care);*

- Oncology patients with resections of primary colorectal cancer whose preoperative evaluation by a managing physician includes examination of the entire colon (examination of the entire colon is a desirable process of care in this situation);† and

- Cardiovascular patients with principal discharge diagnoses of congestive heart failure having documented etiology (documentation of etiology is a desirable process of care).‡

---

* These data are generated by applying the following IMSystem indicator: *Trauma patients with blood pressure, pulse, and respiration documented on arrival and at least hourly for three hours or until emergency department disposition, whichever is earlier.*
† These data are generated by applying the following IMSystem indicator: *Patients with resections of primary colorectal cancer whose preoperative evaluation, by a managing physician, includes examination of the entire colon.*
‡ These data are generated by applying the following IMSystem indicator: *Patients with principal discharge diagnosis of congestive heart failure having a documented etiology.*

Clinical performance data that quantify undesirable outcomes include the following:

- Intrahospital mortality of cardiovascular patients undergoing isolated coronary artery bypass graft surgery, undergoing percutaneous transluminal coronary angioplasty, or with a principal diagnosis of AMI (death is an undesirable outcome);* and
- Intrahospital mortality of trauma patients with a systolic blood pressure of less than 70 mm Hg anytime within two hours of emergency department arrival who did not undergo a laparotomy or thoracotomy (death is an undesirable outcome).†

Clinical Performance Data Information Set

A basic package of information that provides a frame of reference is useful in beginning to interpret clinical performance data. The Joint Commission's IMSystem indicator information sets (also called indicator information forms) are one approach to giving interpreters a context for beginning to make sense of clinical performance data (Figure 2; see pages 16–20). The basic information contained in these sets includes the:

- indicator data focus;
- indicator statement;
- indicator objectives and suggested applications;
- terminology;

---

* These data are generated by applying the following IMSystem indicator: *Intrahospital mortality of cardiovascular patients undergoing isolated coronary artery bypass graft surgery, undergoing percutaneous transluminal angioplasty, or with a principal diagnosis of acute myocardial infarction.*

† These data are generated by applying the following IMSystem indicator: *Intrahospital mortality or trauma patients with a systolic blood pressure of less than 70 mm Hg anytime within two hours of emergency department arrival who did not undergo a laparotomy or thoracotomy.*

- data collection information;
- flow logic; and
- selected references.

The *indicator data focus* is the simplest expression of the intent behind each indicator and its data. It often, but not always, clarifies which dimensions of performance (for example, timeliness) are undergoing measurement. Consider, for example, the following indicator:

> *Trauma patients undergoing selected neurosurgical,*
> *orthopedic, or abdominal surgical procedures: time from*
> *emergency department arrival to procedure.**

Its indicator data focus is:

> *Timeliness of surgical intervention for selected head,*
> *orthopedic, or abdominal injuries.*

Knowing this small piece of information (the indicator focus) enables interpreters to make sense of data (described at the beginning of this chapter) on a hospital's mean time of 66 minutes from arrival in the emergency department to anesthesia induction for patients with specified injuries. Interpreters can deduce that the focus of these indicator data is timeliness with respect to surgical intervention. Timeliness means the degree to which a surgical procedure is provided to a patient at the most beneficial or necessary time.

Consider also the following indicator:

> *Comatose trauma patients with selected intracranial*
> *injuries discharged from the emergency department prior*
> *to endotracheal intubation or cricothyrotomy.†*

Its indicator data focus is:

> *Airway management of comatose trauma patients.*

---

* These data are generated by applying the following IMSystem indicator: *Trauma patients undergoing selected neurosurgical, orthopedic, or abdominal surgical procedures: time from emergency department arrival to induction of anesthesia.*

† These data are generated by applying the following Joint Commission IMSystem indicator: *Comatose trauma patients with selected intracranial injuries discharged from the emergency department prior to endotracheal intubation or cricothyrotomy.*

The indicator data focus enables interpreters to make sense of data in the example at the beginning of this chapter (nine intubated patients, one patient with a cricothyrotomy, and one nonintubated patient with Glasgow Coma Scale scores of less than eight discharged from the emergency department). The indicator data focus concerns proper airway management for comatose patients with selected head injuries.

The *indicator statement* clearly sets forth the population and the process, activity, event, or outcome undergoing measurement. Indicator statements include the following:

> *Patients undergoing treatment for primary cancer of the female breast, lung, or colon/rectum having stage of tumor designated by a managing physician;* and
>
> *Patients with principal discharge diagnosis of congestive heart failure having documented etiology.*[†]

In the first example, the population consists of patients undergoing treatment for primary cancer of the female breast, lung, or colon/rectum; the activity undergoing measurement is designation of the patient's stage of tumor by a managing physician. In the second example, the population consists of patients with a principal discharge diagnosis of congestive heart failure; the event undergoing measurement is documenting the etiology of the congestive heart failure in the patient record.

Indicator objectives and suggested applications contain a wealth of information about the indicator and its data, such as the:

- rationale for measuring the process, activity, event, or outcome;

---

* These data are generated by applying the following IMSystem indicator: *Patients with resections of primary colorectal cancer whose preoperative evaluation, by a managing physician, includes examination of the entire colon.*

† These data are generated by applying the following IMSystem indicator: *Patients with principal discharge diagnosis of congestive heart failure having a documented etiology.*

- type of indicator—process versus outcome;
- type of indicator—desirable versus undesirable;
- type of indicator—continuous variable versus discrete variable;
- way in which indicator data express information, either about many events or individual events; and
- list of patient-based and non-patient-based (that is, practitioner-based or organization-based) factors that may influence indicator data and help organizations make sense of their data.

The rationale behind each indicator and its data is directly related to the strength of the data, explored in Chapter Five. Underlying factors help organizations and clinicians diagnose undesirable variation in clinical performance data. This subject is described in Chapter Eight.

Flow logic refers to the algorithm designed to collect and assemble required data elements to produce the desired indicator data. The flow logic is not the logic of the indicator itself, but of the data collection and assembly process. The approach used by the Joint Commission's IMSystem is described in detail elsewhere.[6] The *Selected References* section of the Performance Data Form provides interpreters with information sources that support indicator rationales.

Summary Observations

Studying important characteristics of clinical performance is the first step in beginning to make sense of the data. There are three points to remember in studying data characteristics:

1. Clinical performance data and their parent indicators are inextricably linked. Making sense of clinical performance data requires knowing the characteristics of the indicator that generated the data.

2. Clinical performance data measure

- one or more dimensions of performance;
- patient health outcomes or patient care processes;
- sentinel events or aggregate performance data; and
- desirable or undesirable outcomes or processes.

Clinical performance data may be reported as either continuous variable data or discrete variable (attribute) data.

3. An indicator information set is a useful package of information that provides a frame of reference for beginning to interpret clinical performance data. The Joint Commission's IMSystem indicator data information set is one such package. It includes the indicator data focus, indicator statement, indicator objectives and suggested applications, terminology, data collection information, flow logic, and selected references.

References

1.　Joint Commission on Accreditation of Healthcare Organizations: *1995 Accreditation Manual for Hospitals.* Oakbrook Terrace, IL: JCAHO, 1994, p 30.

2.　Joint Commission on Accreditation of Healthcare Organizations: *The Measurement Mandate.* Oakbrook Terrace, IL: JCAHO, 1993, pp 67–93.

3.　Joint Commission on Accreditation of Healthcare Organizations: *Lexikon: Dictionary of Health Care Terms, Organizations, and Acronyms for the Era of Reform.* Oakbrook Terrace, IL: JCAHO, 1994, p 579.

4.　Ibid, pp 132–145.

5.　Rowntree D: *Statistics Without Tears: A Primer for Non-mathematicians.* New York: Charles Scribner's Sons, 1981, pp 28–34.

6.　Joint Commission on Accreditation of Healthcare Organizations: *The Measurement Mandate.* Oakbrook Terrace, IL: JCAHO, 1993, pp 149–159.

CHAPTER FIVE

Evaluating the Strength of Clinical Performance Data

The basis for developing sound information lies in strong clinical performance data. Data strength is defined as the degree to which the data demonstrate six important attributes listed here:

- Clinical relevance;
- Range of health care processes and outcomes addressed by clinical performance data;
- Reliability;
- Validity;
- Variation; and
- Degree to which health care providers have control over processes and outcomes measured.

The field of evaluating these attributes to determine data strength is in its infancy. One observer opines that no available measures of performance or quality can successfully "pass" tests of reliability, validity, and other attributes.[1] Awareness about strength-of-data issues is growing, and a small number of progressive organizations are successfully tackling strength-of-data issues.

The Joint Commission, for instance, has a seven-year track record in emphasizing the need to provide data users with strong data, particularly data whose reliability and validity are quantified.

The Joint Commission's findings during beta field testing of its performance indicators have formed the centerpiece of debate as to whether beta indicators should be retained as is, retained and modified, or dropped.

The work of the Joint Commission in developing strong clinical performance data is, however, the exception. The great mass of clinical performance data beginning to reach the public domain has never been subjected to reliability, validity, or any other type of testing to determine strength.

One observer, for instance, points out that there are a growing number of companies in the business of producing physician performance data. These data measure the performance of physicians, but at present nobody is monitoring the performance of the data suppliers. The observer states that "although most such vendors recommend that their reports be used only anonymously and only for the information of the profiled physicians themselves, the potential for abuse is great....If data are used in making such critical professional decisions as whether to grant clinical privileges or recertification, then *the data must be clinically meaningful [relevant] and highly reliable*" (italics added for emphasis).[2]

Data interpreters must exercise extreme caution at this early stage of data interpretation because the performance information's accuracy is directly related to the corresponding data's strength. Performance data that lack acceptable degrees of relevance, reliability, validity, and variation (among other attributes) have the potential to produce irrelevant information (a waste of resources) or, worse, serious misinformation that can contribute to poor decisions.

Relevance of Clinical Performance Data

The strength of a given set of clinical performance data depends on whether the data are relevant to health care providers. *Relevance* is the degree to which clinical performance data relate to what organizations do—that is, functions or processes—and the relative importance of these functions or processes.

The relevance of clinical performance data, however, lies in the eye of the beholder. A medical risk-management company, for instance, may be interested in clinical performance data on acute myocardial infarction, head trauma, pulmonary embolism, and antibiotic treatment of complex infections because these diagnoses and conditions (and their associated processes and outcomes) are involved in the most costly malpractice claims against physicians insured by that company.[3] In this example, management of patients with a specified high-risk diagnosis, such as potential or confirmed acute myocardial infarction, is a process of care; its importance is based on its involvement in costly claims.

A health maintenance organization may be interested in data pertaining to preventive health care practices, such as immunizations for children and mammography examinations for women over age 40. It may also be interested in data on the efficiency of health services delivery, measured by primary care physicians referring patients to specialists and length of patients' hospital stays, subcategorized by physician.[4] A hospital-accrediting body may be interested in data pertaining to services traditionally provided in the hospital setting, such as perioperative (anesthesia and surgical) care, obstetrical care, and trauma care.[5]

Clinical performance data that address irrelevant or marginally relevant issues will not be as useful in decision making no matter how strong their other attributes, such as reliability, may be. Producing data that are truly meaningful to users is why parties interested in using clinical performance data should be intimately involved in developing the indicators that are used to generate the data.[6] The data will have relevance because the questions posed by indicator developers and framed with indicators have relevance.

An Approach to Assessing Indicator Data Relevance

The relevance of indicator data may be assessed by directly questioning users. This approach was used by the Joint Commission, which asked representatives from beta-testing hospitals about their perception of the relevance of each indicator they tested. Joint Commission staff obtained these assessments through a mail survey and follow-up phone calls conducted in November and December, 1993, for cardiovascular, oncology, and trauma care indicators. Individual indicator assessment forms were distributed to beta liaisons at each test hospital, who were asked to distribute the survey to all hospital staff (especially physicians) who played a key role in the indicator-testing project.

Consider, for instance, the following two trauma care beta indicators:

> *Trauma patients with diagnosis of laceration of the liver or spleen, requiring surgery, undergoing laparotomy greater than two hours after emergency department arrival, subcategorized by pediatric or adult patients;* *
> and
> *Trauma patients with prehospital emergency medical services scene times of greater than 20 minutes.*†

Beta-testing hospital personnel were asked for each indicator, "Is this indicator relevant to the patient care services in my hospital?" For TR-7, the median response value was 4.45 on a scale of 1.0 (strongly disagree) to 5.0 (strongly agree). For TR-1, the median response was 3.96.

These measurements of relevance from individuals who actually used the indicators were considered by Joint Commission task forces in deciding how to improve individual indicators and, ultimately, which beta indicators would be recommended for inclusion in the IMSystem pool of indicators.

A useful way to gauge the relevance of performance data is to

---

* This indicator was developed by the Joint Commission Trauma Care Task Force for Indicator Development and selected in a revised form for inclusion in the IMSystem.

† This indicator was developed by the Joint Commission Trauma Care Task Force for Indicator Development but was not selected for inclusion in the IMSystem.

assess the degree to which data address, from the perspective of the interpreters, high-volume, high-risk, problem-prone, and/or high-cost patient care processes or patient health outcomes. A fifth category is the degree to which data address high-visibility processes and outcomes, typically identified by the media. Data that address a combination of these categories (for example, a process that is both high volume and problem prone, or an outcome that is high cost, high visibility, and high risk) would have higher degrees of relevance.

High volume. *High volume* means patient care processes that are performed frequently, affect large numbers of patients, or both. In this category, organizations focus on processes that affect populations of people, rather than individuals, so that improvements have broad impact. Diagnostic testing in hospitals, for example, is a high-volume function because most patients receive some type of laboratory test, diagnostic imaging procedure, or both, during hospitalization. Immunizations, subcategorized by type (for example, measles/mumps/rubella, oral polio), mammography screening, Pap smear screening, cesarean delivery, and vaginal birth after cesarean delivery are high-volume processes; improvements in these processes will affect large patient populations.

High volume also refers to patient health outcomes that occur frequently, affect large numbers of patients, or both. Survival following coronary artery bypass graft surgery, lung cancer mortality, breast cancer mortality, and mortality of Medicare patients with acute myocardial infarction within 30 days of hospital admission are examples of high-volume outcomes. Improvements in these outcomes will affect relatively large patient populations.

High risk. *High risk* means three categories of patient care processes: processes that are needed but not performed; "risky" processes that are performed but not needed; and processes that are needed and performed, but performed poorly. High-risk processes expose patients to a greater chance of undesirable outcomes.

An example of a process that is indicated but not performed is failing to perform an abdominal ultrasound on an eight-week pregnant patient who comes to the emergency department complaining of abdominal pain. The patient's obstetrician refuses to "waste resources" on the ultrasound examination because ectopic pregnancy had been ruled out during a physical examination the day before. Or, in another case, sending a self-paying (noninsured) patient with possible symptoms of cardiac ischemic disease home from the emergency department, with the potential result of a preventable out-of-hospital cardiac arrest.

An example of a risky process that is performed when it is not needed is admitting a nonmorbid adult patient with chickenpox to a university hospital as a teaching case. A lack of beds results in the patient being assigned to the only available isolation bed in the hospital, which is on the obstetrics ward. The patient is wheeled through the neonatal unit to the available isolation bed where she stays for an hour or two before the mistake is noted. In this example, the wrong decision to admit can result in serious illness for the newborns exposed to chickenpox.

An example of a process that is needed but is performed poorly is inappropriate delay in assessing and moving a patient with a serious injury (such as a lacerated spleen) or a serious illness (such as appendicitis) from the emergency department to an operating room for necessary surgical intervention. Inappropriate delays of this kind can result in an undesirable outcome (such as loss of blood from a lacerated spleen or ruptured appendix) for the patient, the patient's family, the clinicians caring for the patient, and the organization providing the care.

High-risk processes may also be complex new procedures that are inherently risky because the services being provided may never have been performed before or have been performed so few times that their safety and efficacy remain under investigation. Other high-risk processes may be ones that are performed for patients whose preexisting characteristics may influence the outcomes. The process may be carried out perfectly, but a desired outcome may be impossible to achieve because of characteristics specific to the patient. For instance, anesthetic services carry a high degree of risk if they are performed for patients with severe systemic disease that is a constant threat to life (American Society of Anesthesiologists-Physical Status Class 4).

Problem prone. *Problem prone* means processes that have produced problems for patients, their families, health care providers, and purchasers. These processes tend to be difficult to accomplish for two reasons:

- The need for interlinked organizational systems to work in synchrony to achieve desired objectives is not adequately met; or

- Basic, routinely relied-on processes and systems are operating poorly (the output of these processes and systems is chaotic and unpredictable).

Lack of synchrony can affect any process used to assess and stabilize patients with life-threatening emergencies. Emergencies usually require the synchronized input of multiple organizational systems within a short period of time to achieve acceptable patient outcomes. A failure anywhere in a system, subsystem, or process can result in undesirable outcomes, including preventable death.

Unpredictable outputs can affect any process linked to availability of clinical data in the patient record. When important data are unavailable to caregivers, patient care can suffer. Medical records that are missing pathology reports for patients undergoing resections for cancer, for instance, can increase the possibility that a physician will select an inappropriate or inadequate treatment. Unavailable test results, such as estrogen receptor diagnostic analysis results for patients with Stage II or greater primary breast cancer, may affect treatment decisions, cancer recurrence, and patient survival. In each of these examples, the process(es) for including important data in patient records is operating poorly.

High cost. *High cost* means that total expenses for performing a process or achieving an outcome are elevated by one of two criteria. Either the absolute cost is elevated or the cost is elevated compared to some point. An elevated absolute cost might be $20,000 (including physician and hospital fees) incurred by a patient or other purchaser for receiving a specified procedure.

Costs may be elevated when compared to, for example, the mean cost for a group or an area, or the lowest cost available among a group or in an area. For instance, the price charged by hospitals in St Louis for cataract removal varies from a high of $5,112 to a low of $915 (average fee, $2,744), according to one source. The price charged by ophthalmologists in St Louis varies from a high of $3,266 to a low of $1,400 (average fee, $2,265). The average negotiated managed-care payment for cataract removal among the same group of ophthalmologists is $1,964. Medicare's maximum payment to this group of physicians was $1,082.[7]

Or, for example, the prices for performing a diagnostic test, such as measuring prostate-specific antigen (PSA) in the blood, may vary from a high of $114 to a low of $10 (average fee, $68).[8] The difference between high and low prices is 1,040%. Thus, the absolute cost to society of performing a procedure can be quite high if that procedure is high cost *and* high volume. Data that identify procedures or outcomes that are high cost possess a high degree of relevance for many stakeholders in health care today.

High visibility. *High visibility* means processes or outcomes thrust into the limelight by the media. The processes and outcomes of interest may be related to well-known figures such as people holding or running for political office. Media stories about individuals and their health care experiences have the potential to expose readers to copious information, such as the increased public awareness and knowledge of trauma care following the intense media coverage of the care provided after the 1981 presidential assassination attempt. The public's awareness and knowledge of substance abuse was increased from the efforts of at least two former First Ladies and the processes and outcomes of care for surgically separating the Lakeberg conjoined (Siamese) twins received detailed coverage. Clinical performance data rapidly acquire a high degree of relevance to many parties when intimate details of care processes and outcomes become public knowledge.

Range of Health Care Processes and Outcomes Addressed by Clinical Performance Data

A broad range of health care processes and outcomes must be addressed by clinical performance data for at least two important reasons. First, *data users must invest improvement resources where they will do the most good, not just some good.* Data from a broad range of processes or outcomes will provide the input necessary to determine where resources should be directed.[9]

For instance, an organization's performance data for cardiovascular processes and outcomes are showing general improvement, whereas performance data from trauma processes and outcomes are showing increasing undesirable variation. The organization could invest further resources into thriving clinical areas to make them even better, or the organization could invest resources into troublesome areas. The availability of data that address a broad range of clinical areas, processes, and outcomes affords organizations the opportunity to better meet patient needs.

Second, *a range of health care processes and outcomes must be addressed by clinical performance data so that data users avoid causing (or failing to prevent) harm elsewhere in the organization.* There is a real danger in basing improvement activities on a limited set of measurement data. These data may, perhaps unintentionally, result in poorer performance elsewhere in the organization. For example, in an organization that bases its improvement activities on a limited set of performance data, one clinical area in the organization is thriving. It produces abundant performance data that compel organizational leadership to allocate additional resources to improvements in that clinical area. Another clinical area in the same organization, however, is strapped for resources but has few measurements to demonstrate its needs. By allocating resources according to a limited set of data, the organization may inadvertently be contributing to poor performance elsewhere in the organization.

Reliability of Clinical Performance Data

Demonstration that clinical performance data can reliably quantify processes or outcomes of care is an essential attribute of an effective performance measurement system; however, error-free measurement is never attained in any area of scientific investigation because *unreliability* is always present to at least a limited extent.[10, 11] Nevertheless, an acceptable level of reliability should be present if data are to provide a relatively accurate representation of the process or outcome undergoing measurement.

What is data reliability? *Data reliability* is the extent to which data results are consistent across repeated measurements of the same phenomenon by different measurers or at different times by the same measurers. The phenomenon must not have changed in the interval between measurements.[10]

Data reliability can pose many problems in performance measurement. For instance, the following indicator requires a very specific data element: *Glasgow Coma Scale (GCS) score upon arrival of a trauma patient to the emergency department.* Suppose that an abstractor cannot readily locate the GCS in patient records. Instead, he or she uses the GCS found on patients' prehospital emergency medical services ambulance run sheets or intensive care unit flow sheets. Suppose that another abstractor enters patients' trauma scores, even though trauma scores and GCS scores are different and noninterchangeable measures. These practices lead to collecting inconsistent and, therefore, unreliable data, which would not accurately represent the concept they are supposed to be measuring.

Another indicator requires the following data element: *time that patients arrive at the emergency department.* Suppose that a precise definition for this time—such as the time that a patient is first assessed by clinical staff—is not provided, or is provided but not heeded by individuals abstracting the data element from emergency department patient records. This ambiguity leads to some abstractors recording the time that the ambulance arrived at the emergency department, others recording the time that the patient was registered by the emergency department, and still others reporting the time that a caregiver first treated the patient or first wrote something in the patient record. Again, it is not difficult to understand the potential inaccuracy and unreliability of the collected data.

Data reliability has been described as a measure of the degree to which data generated by an individual indicator are free from *random error.*[10] Random error in data is caused by chance factors that confound the measurement of processes and outcomes. The amount of random error is inversely related to the indicator's degree of reliability. The effects of random error are totally unsystematic. In other words, the lower the amount of random error present in an indicator's data, the more reliable is the indicator. Examples of random error include human documentation errors and ambiguities in defining data elements.

Reliability Testing

There are four basic methods for estimating the reliability of clinical performance data:

- Retest method;
- Alternative-form method;
- Split-halves method; and
- Internal consistency method.

The retest method, one of the easiest ways to estimate the reliability of clinical performance data, involves performing the same measurement after a period of time. The Joint Commission used an adaptation of this approach in beta testing the reliability of its clinical performance indicators and data. The Joint Commission's approach is briefly described below; see Chapter Six and other sources in the "References" section for a full treatment of reliability testing.[10]

An Approach to Assessing Data Reliability

The retest method was used to assess the reliability of the data generated by Joint Commission indicator sets for cardiovascular care, oncology care, and trauma care (November 1992 through May 1993). Pairs of highly trained Joint Commission staff traveled to beta-testing hospitals selected by a Joint Commission biostatistician, through a stratified random sampling procedure, from among several hundred accredited U.S. hospitals involved in the beta-testing process. Strata were based on four geographic regions, three bed sizes (200, 200 to 400, and 400 plus), and urban versus rural.

Joint Commission staff reabstracted patient records, previously identified by a sampling procedure, in which indicator events had occurred or were at risk of occurring, according to data already transmitted to the Joint Commission by the beta test hospitals. A total of 75 hospitals were visited; data were collected at 54 sites for trauma care indicators, 58 sites for oncology care indicators, and 64 sites for cardiovascular care indicators.

Reliability testing was made up of two components: evaluating the integrity of individual data elements (data reliability) and determining the accuracy and consistency of identifying indicator events (indicator reliability) across beta test sites. In the latter case, reliability was quantified as the proportion of the total number of cases correctly categorized as indicator-identified records (true positives) plus those eligible only for the denominator population (true negatives), divided by the total number of cases reabstracted. See *The Measurement Mandate* for an in-depth treatment of the indicator categories developed and used by the Joint Commission (see Table 4, page 77).[12]

Cases that did not qualify for a particular indicator's denominator population (ineligible cases) were excluded from the calculation if these cases were categorized as ineligible by *both* the hospital abstractors and the Joint Commission reabstractors. False-positive cases (indicator occurrences transmitted by the beta test site that were found to be nonevents when reabstracted by Joint

TABLE 4 Definitions of Indicator Categories

Category 1   means there are insufficient data to determine whether the record is a member of the population referenced by the indicator (the denominator population). Eligibility of the case for inclusion in the indicator occurrence rate is undetermined because key data elements that determine if the case meets criteria for consideration are missing from the database.

Category 2   means the record is not a member of the denominator population referenced by the indicator. The record is therefore ineligible because sufficient data elements are in the database to determine that the case does not meet the criteria for the specified indicator.

Category 3   means the record is a member of the reference (denominator) population but more data are needed to fully classify the record. The record has potential numerator eligibility because sufficient data elements are present to determine that the case is in the denominator, but there are insufficient data to determine if the case is an indicator event.

Category 4   means the record is a member of the reference (denominator) population for the indicator, but it lacks the outcome characteristics that were measured, and it therefore is not an indicator event; the case is a denominator case only. The record has an eligible denominator, meaning sufficient data are present to determine that the case belongs in the denominator.

Category 5   means the record is a member of the indicator reference population and has the characteristics that were measured by the indicator (numerator as well as denominator case). This record is an indicator-identified case, meaning that sufficient data are present to determine that the case meets the criteria for an indicator event.

Source: Joint Commission on Accreditation of Healthcare Organizations: *The Measurement Mandate.* Oakbrook Terrace, IL: JCAHO, 1993, p 157.

Commission staff) and false-negative cases (indicator nonevents transmitted by the beta test site that were found to be events upon reabstraction) were also identified and categorized.

Examples of three indicators' reliability measurements are presented below. These measurements include the percentage of cases categorized the same by the test site and the Joint Commission, the percentage of false positives, and the percentage of false negatives.

The first example involves the following beta cardiovascular indicator:

> *Intrahospital mortality of patients undergoing isolated coronary artery bypass graft (CABG) procedures, subcategorized by initial and subsequent CABG procedures, by emergent or nonemergent clinical status, and by postoperative day and intrahospital location of death.**

Joint Commission personnel reabstracted 216 cases. Of these 216 cases, 215 (99.5%) were categorized the same by the test site and the Joint Commission reabstractors. There were no false-positive cases and no false-negative cases.

The second example involves the following beta oncology indicator:

> *Patients undergoing pulmonary resection for primary lung cancer with postoperative complication of empyema, bronchopleural fistula, reoperation for postoperative bleeding, mechanical ventilation greater than five days postoperatively, or intrahospital death.†*

Joint Commission personnel reabstracted 157 cases. Of these 157 cases, 148 (94.3%) were categorized the same by the test site and

---

* This indicator was developed by the Joint Commission Cardiovascular Care Task Force for Indicator Development and was selected in a revised form for inclusion in the IMSystem.

† This indicator was developed by the Joint Commission Oncology Care Task Force for Indicator Development but was not selected for inclusion in the IMSystem.

the Joint Commission reabstractors. There were 2.9% false-positive cases and no false-negative cases.

The third example involves the following beta trauma indicator:

*Trauma patients transferred from initial receiving hospital to another acute care facility within six hours from emergency department (ED) arrival to ED departure.**

Joint Commission personnel reabstracted 125 cases. Of these 125 cases, 113 (90.4%) were categorized the same by the test site and the Joint Commission reabstractors. There were 2.7% false-positive cases and 4.4% false-negative cases.

Reliability was also examined at the level of individual data elements, such as specific times. For instance, of 1,184 cases in which both the hospital abstractor and the Joint Commission reabstractor had complete information about emergency department patient arrival time, there was *agreement* (to the exact minute) between the hospital abstractor and the Joint Commission reabstractor in 62.2% of cases. Of the 37.8% of cases in which there was *disagreement* in time, the discrepancy was less than 10 minutes in two thirds of the cases.

What to Do with Reliability Data

Interpreters must make judgments as to what is an acceptable level of indicator and data reliability. Reliability scores higher than 80% are desirable. Lower reliability scores mean that a large number of false positives and false negatives exist. False positives inflate occurrence rates and overstate the need for an organization's response to data. False negatives result in artificially low indicator rates that may fail to trigger needed organization or clinician response.

In general, as reliability falls off, the data's usefulness tends to decline. One notable exception is when performance issues, such as a high-risk or high-visibility process of care, become highly relevant

---

* This indicator was developed by the Joint Commission Trauma Care Task Force for Indicator Development but was not selected for inclusion in the IMSystem.

to organizations. The more important an issue becomes, the more organizations may choose to tolerate lower performance data reliability. They understand that accepting a lower level of reliability requires more assessment of the performance issue before action is taken.

Validity of Clinical Performance Data

Clinical performance data must be more than reliable if they are to provide an accurate representation of the performance dimension they are measuring. Data must also be valid. What, then, is data validity?

Data validity is the extent to which an indicator and its data measure only what they were intended to measure.[13, 14] In performance measurement, indicators are developed and applied because people want tools that can provide answers to their questions about performance. Consider the indicator that measures the appropriateness with which vital signs are assessed by staff caring for seriously or potentially seriously injured trauma patients. Patients, purchasers, and health care providers are interested in the data produced by this indicator because the data can tell them whether good (appropriate, or correct) care is being provided for this group of patients. Once the data are collected, the validity question is: Do the data in fact measure the degree to which appropriate care is being provided or do the data measure something else?

Carrying this example further, consider a hospital whose rate for this indicator is very low. The low rate triggers in-depth evaluation of the process of care. First, the hospital determines that the data are, in fact, reliable, meaning that frequent vital signs are *not* recorded in the patient records. When clinical staff are interviewed about this, they say that they take vital signs with great frequency but do not have time to document them in patient records. The hospital cries foul because, from its perspective, the indicator and its data are not measuring only what they were intended to measure. Good care *is* being provided, according to the hospital, but the indicator data do not reflect this. The data, from the perspective of the hospital, are invalid for the purpose for which they are being used.

Or instead of finding that frequent vital signs were missing from the patient records, the hospital finds that frequent vital signs were almost always present but, for some reason, abstractors could not locate them. This situation characterizes what is meant by a false-positive case. The hospital again cries foul because, from its perspective, the indicator and its data have failed to measure what they were intended to measure. Performance of vital signs, they argue, is very good (they can prove it), but the data do not accurately reflect this fact.

A third example of data validity issues also involves a hospital with a low indicator rate for obtaining frequent vital signs on trauma patients. The hospital further investigates the process of care, only to be notified by emergency department staff that obtaining at least hourly vital signs on all patients, even those with minor abrasions, is ridiculous. From the perspective of the emergency department staff, the data are invalid for determining whether appropriate care is being provided. Once emergency department staff become aware that the data measure the appropriateness with which care is provided to the most seriously or potentially seriously injured trauma patients, they usually readily agree that a low indicator rate for this process of care represents a serious opportunity for improvement.

Important Types of Validity

There are four major types of validity. *Face validity* reflects the extent to which a performance measure and its data make intuitive sense and seem relevant and appropriate to experts in a clinical area. Face validity can be assessed, for instance, through determining degrees of consensus among various stakeholders or through peer review.

Construct validity is the extent to which a performance measure and its data quantify what they were designed to quantify. The performance measure and its data can be evaluated in comparison to some "gold standard" performance measure, if one exists.

Convergent validity involves correlations among two or more measures, such as indicators or their data, of a concept. Convergent validity does not assume that one measure is a gold standard against which other measures should be evaluated.

Scientific validity is the degree to which a demonstrable, causal relationship exists between a process and the outcomes of the process. It is related to predictive validity since causal relationships would predict specific outcomes.

An Approach to Validation Testing

Validation testing of a method or tool may be viewed as the process of establishing that the method or tool is sound. According to Cronbach, "validity is subjective, rather than objective; the plausibility of the conclusion is what counts."[15]

The Joint Commission used one approach to assessing indicator data validity by asking representatives from beta test sites the five following questions:

- Does a particular indicator and its data raise good questions about organizational performance?
- Does a particular indicator and its data identify opportunities for improving organizational performance?
- Do organizations take action to improve performance based on indicator data?
- Do these actions result in changes in organizational processes, outcomes, or both?
- Do indicators and their data benefit the organization?

These assessments were obtained through a mail survey conducted in November and December, 1993, for cardiovascular, oncology, and trauma care indicators. Individual indicator assessment forms were distributed to beta liaisons at each test hospital, who were asked to distribute the survey to all hospital staff (especially physicians) *who played a key role in the indicator-testing project.*

The set of nine cardiovascular care beta indicators had a survey response rate of 75%. Validity-testing data showed that the majority of respondents believed that indicators CV-6, CV-7, CV-8, and CV-9 were best able to identify opportunities to improve patient care.* For example, approximately 50% of respondents rated highly the following indicator:

Patients admitted for acute myocardial infarction (AMI), rule-out AMI, or unstable angina who have a discharge diagnosis of AMI...,

but only approximately 25% of respondents rated highly the following indicator (CV-1):

Intrahospital mortality of patients undergoing isolated coronary artery bypass graft procedures...

Certain indicators were also more likely to trigger action within beta test sites, particularly indicators CV-8 and CV-9. The data produced by these two indicators triggered action in approximately one-third of beta test sites, according to respondents.

What to Do with Validity Data

Interpreters must decide what is an acceptable level of indicator and data validity, with high validity being more desirable. The data's usefulness is directly related to how valid they are in the eyes of users.

---

* CV-6: *Intrahospital mortality of patients with principal discharge diagnosis of acute myocardial infarction, subcategorized by history of previous infarction, age, and intrahospital location of death;*
CV-7: *Patients admitted for acute myocardial infarction (AMI), rule-out AMI, or unstable angina who have a discharge diagnosis of AMI, subcategorized by admission to an intensive care unit, a monitored bed, or an unmonitored bed;*
CV-8: *Patients with principal discharge diagnosis of congestive heart failure (CHF) with documented etiology and chest x-ray substantiation of CHF;*
CV-9: *Patients with a principal discharge diagnosis of congestive heart failure (CHF) with at least two determinations of patient weight and of serum sodium, potassium, blood urea nitrogen, and creatinine levels.*

Data Reliability and Validity

Data reliability and validity are distinct, but interlinked, attributes that are present in varying degrees. Unreliable data will almost always be invalid data. Reliable data, however, may not necessarily be valid data for a particular purpose. Although an indicator's data elements may be collected with a high rate of consistency, this does not necessarily mean those elements will meet users' intentions and needs.

Variation in Clinical Performance Data

Clinical performance data will always show some degree of variation, but as the amount of variation increases, there is frequently a greater opportunity to identify performance improvement opportunities. Thus, variation is an extremely important attribute of strong clinical performance data. Variation is addressed in this section as a prelude to the full discussion in Chapter Seven.

Variation in data has two distinct meanings. First, it means the *spread,* or *dispersion*, of data around an average (mean, median) over time. Second, it refers to the *discrepancy*, or *deviation*, between a data set's average value and the established (well-accepted) average for the process or outcome undergoing measurement. These two definitions drive two separate approaches to assessing the variation in a given set of data.

First Approach to Assessing Variation in Data

The following indicator provides an example of variation in data viewed as the spread of data around an average:

> *Patients admitted for acute myocardial infarction (AMI), rule-out AMI, or unstable angina who have a discharge diagnosis of AMI.**

---

* This indicator was developed by the Joint Commission Cardiovascular Care Task Force for Indicator Development and was selected for inclusion in the IMSystem.

The interquartile range (dividing the distribution's spread into four equal parts; see Chapter Six) was calculated as the measure of spread for this indicator's data set. The interquartile range was from 30.2% (Q1) to 74.2% (Q3), according to Joint Commission beta test site data. This means that 25% of test site hospitals had rates of less than 30.2%, and 75% of hospitals had rates of less than 74.2%. The median indicator rate for the group of test site hospitals was 46.4%. An interquartile range of between 30.2% and 74.2% is relatively wide, suggesting that there are opportunities to improve the process measured by the indicator data.

Compare that example to the variation observed for the following indicator:

> *Trauma patients transferred from initial receiving*
> *hospital to another acute care facility within six hours*
> *from emergency department (ED) arrival to ED*
> *departure.**

The interquartile range for these data was 97.0% (Q1) to 100% (Q3), according to Joint Commission beta test site data. This interquartile range (97% to 100%) is very narrow, suggesting that opportunities to improve this particular process—that is, transferring trauma patients within a six-hour time frame—are probably limited.

Second Approach to Assessing Variation in Data

The following indicator provides an example of variation as the discrepancy between a data set's average value and an established (well-accepted) value:

> *Trauma patients who had their blood pressure, pulse*
> *rate, respiratory rate, and Glasgow Coma Scale score*
> *documented in the emergency department record on*
> *arrival and at least hourly until inpatient admission to*

---

* This indicator was developed by the Joint Commission Trauma Care Task Force for Indicator Development but was not selected for inclusion in the IMSystem.

> *an operating room or intensive care unit, death, or*
> *transfer to another care facility.**

The median hospital indicator rate for this process of care was 9.7%, according to Joint Commission beta test site data. (Analysis of the data showed that the Glasgow Coma Scale was not being used 100% of the time, which contributed to the relatively low median rate of 9.7% observed for this indicator.) The median hospital indicator rate for monitoring this group of patients (seriously injured or potentially seriously injured) should approach 100%. The discrepancy between 9.7% (measured value) and 100% (established value) is quite large, suggesting that there are probably many opportunities to improve monitoring within this group of trauma patients in the emergency department.

Compare that example to the indicator previously described about transferring trauma patients within six hours of arrival at the emergency department. The median value for transferring trauma patients within six hours calculated for test site hospitals was 100%. The established average rate for this process is also 100%. The lack of any discrepancy between the observed rate and the established rate suggests that opportunities will be scarce for improving on the transfer of trauma patients within a six-hour time frame. The data strongly suggest that the performance objective has already been met.

Variation in Data Comes in Degrees

Variation in data comes in degrees—that is, some data sets will show more variation than others. There are three general guidelines that assist in interpreting the variation observed in clinical performance data.

First, wider variation in data usually signals more improvement opportunities, while narrower variation in data usually signals fewer

---

* This indicator was developed by the Joint Commission Trauma Care Task Force for Indicator Development and was selected in a revised form for inclusion in the IMSystem.

improvement opportunities. This is shown in Figure 8 (A is wide variation; B is narrow variation; see page 88).[16]

Second, a large discrepancy between a data set's average value and the generally established and well-accepted (that is, desired) average signals more improvement opportunities, and a small or nonexistent discrepancy signals fewer opportunities. This is portrayed in Figure 8C and Figures 8A and 8B (nonexistent discrepancy).

Third, the greatest opportunity for improvement probably comes with data that show both wide variation with respect to their average and their average is displaced from the established and well-accepted (desired) average (Figure 8D). The least opportunity for improvement comes with data that show narrow variation with respect to their average, which is *not* displaced from the established average (Figure 8B).

Approaches to Assessing Variation

The Joint Commission assessed variation in clinical performance data sets by using interquartile range as a measure of the spread of data around the median over time (the first approach described).

A second approach to assessing variation—that is, assessing the discrepancy, or deviation, between a data set's average value and the average for the process or outcome undergoing measurement—was more difficult to carry out. Established and well-accepted average values are available for some processes and outcomes, such as for intrahospital mortality associated with coronary artery bypass surgery or performance of cesarean section. However, established and well-accepted averages are extremely scarce for the vast majority of patient care processes and outcomes, particularly those of an everyday nature. This paucity is a result of the lack of broad-based interest in performance measurement in health care during the twentieth century.

When established averages are scarce, a database-derived average can be used as a starting point; however, this average may not represent the most desired value, only the most commonly encountered value.

FIGURE 8 Possible Distributions in Clinical Performance Data

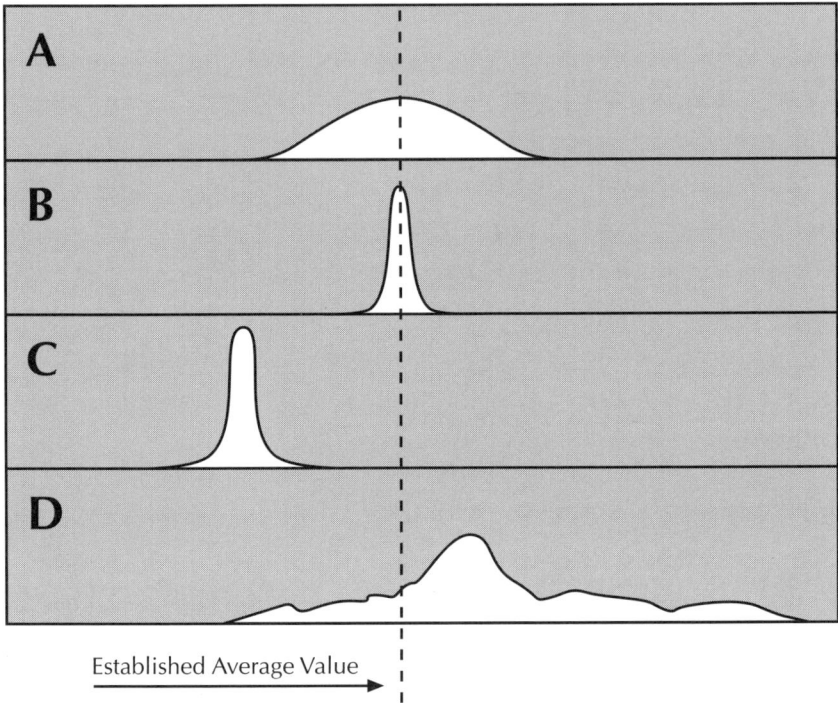

A   Frequency distribution showing very wide variation around an established average value

B   Frequency distribution showing narrow variation around an established average value

C   Frequency distribution showing narrow variation around an average value displaced from the established average value

D   Frequency distribution showing wide variation around an average value displaced from the established average value

Source: Adapted from Deming WE: *The New Economics for Industry, Government, Education*. Cambridge, MA: Massachusetts Institute of Technology Center for Advanced Engineering Study, 1993, pp 82, 130. Used with permission.

This figure shows some of the possible distributions commonly seen in clinical performance data.

What to Do with Variation in Data Measurements

Data interpreters must make judgments as to what is an acceptable degree of variation in data. A high degree of variation in data is desirable because it usually signals more improvement opportunities. This is especially true of data that are widely spread around their average, which is substantially displaced from an established average.

Degree of Provider Control over Measured Processes and Outcomes

The final important attribute of strong data is the degree to which organizations and clinicians actually have control over a process or an outcome undergoing measurement. Without this control, improvement efforts can be both costly and futile.

Consider, for instance, data that measure trauma patients' prehospital emergency medical services scene times.* The length of time emergency medical personnel spend at the scene is an important process linked to outcomes. The condition of critically injured patients frequently deteriorates over time; the more time emergency medical personnel spend at the scene performing various procedures, the greater the chance that this deterioration will occur. Thus, except for problems in patient extrication, trauma patients should be rapidly transported to a hospital where definitive trauma services can be provided.

However, in an emergency medical services system that is independent of a hospital's emergency or trauma services, the hospital and clinicians might understandably question why they should collect and interpret data about a process of care for which they are not accountable and have no power to change, even when opportunities for improvement are clear.

---

* This indicator was developed by the Joint Commission Trauma Care Task Force for Indicator Development but was not selected for inclusion in the IMSystem.

In many cases, individual clinicians may be responsible for outcomes over which they had little control; the outcomes were predominantly influenced by failures in organizational processes or systems. W. Edwards Deming writes:

> Every suit for malpractice in medicine, or in engineering or accounting, implicates the event to a special cause— somebody was at fault. Study with the aid of a bit of knowledge about variation leads to a different conclusion: the event could well have come from the process itself. It could have been built in, guaranteed.[17]

For example, first-year or second-year resident physicians perform some fairly risky procedures in a hospital, unsupervised by more experienced physicians who are not readily available. When an undesirable outcome results from performing such a procedure, blame is typically affixed to the less experienced physician, who may be reprimanded by his or her superiors in the organization and eventually sued for malpractice by the patient and his or her family. People who understand variation, however, will likely conclude that the outcome could have come from the system for supervising inexperienced physicians. Improving the level of supervision for all resident physicians would benefit patients more than severely disciplining physicians who, because they were inadequately supervised, committed judgment or technical errors. Dismissing every resident physician who committed such an error would still not prevent future resident physicians from committing similar errors *as long as the underlying system problem remained unaddressed.*

Striking a Balance Among the Attributes of Data

Probably the most challenging aspect of assessing a data set's strength is to integrate the six main attributes described in this chapter to arrive at an overall assessment of the data set. The challenge comes from these factors: first, there is typically a large amount of information to integrate; second, a data set may be very strong in one attribute, such as validity or relevance, but weak in another, such as reliability or variation; and third, there is currently no appropriate and effective way of assigning weight to each attribute to form an overall assessment.

Approaches to Assessing Overall Strength of Clinical Performance Data

The Joint Commission used two approaches to assess the overall strength of the clinical performance data that emerged from the beta-testing phase of cardiovascular, oncology, and trauma care indicator sets. This assessment was important because indicator data sets' strength determined which field-tested indicators would be included in the IMSystem. Also, strength-of-data attributes guided all the fine-tuning improvements on indicators that made the final cut.

The first approach involved setting a very high priority on actually measuring the various strength-of-data attributes during rigorous field testing of all the indicators developed by the Joint Commission's expert task forces. It is impossible to underestimate the importance of *testing*— that is, *using*—indicators before implementing them. Testing indicators provides the opportunity to actually measure data attributes and then make rational judgments about the data's strength, based on the measurements. Without testing indicators, the strength of data can only be surmised, usually inaccurately.

The second approach involved reconvening the original task forces that had created the indicators, which were field tested by hundreds of voluntary accredited hospitals in the United States. The task forces were charged with studying the strength of data, modifying indicators when necessary to improve strength, and recommending approximately five indicators per task force. All the measurements concerning strength-of-data attributes were presented and hours of discussion among task force members followed. The measurements were ranked after voting by secret ballot. Each task force's chairperson presented the indicators that emerged from this process to representatives of the Joint Commission's Board of Commissioners.

Lessons Learned in Large-Scale Testing and Data Assessment

The testing and data assessment processes were challenging for all parties concerned. Five lessons deserve attention because they reflect important underlying issues and concerns that may arise during these processes.

First, rigorous testing of performance measures with large-scale applicability is a brand-new undertaking in the health care field. The process of testing performance measures requires persistence, patience, and a clear focus on the goal of producing high-quality indicator data.

Second, the actual testing of performance measures often falls into the domain of methodology experts, including information specialists who reabstract patient records, researchers who conduct surveys, and biostatisticians and computer experts who oversee project data collection and aggregation. It is critical during this time that methodology experts and content (clinical) experts not lose touch with each other. Any tendency for one group or the other to become territorial by claiming sole ownership of clinical performance data must be averted. Content and methodology experts bring different assets to the process; their roles must be complementary, not competitive, to produce high-quality clinical performance data.

Third, the length of time required to develop and test clinical performance measures well does not seem to significantly dampen the enthusiasm of the majority of clinical and methodology experts involved in the work. By the end of the Joint Commission's testing process, for instance, most of the content experts embraced data assessment with relish and looked forward to helping interpret clinical performance data generated by the IMSystem.

Fourth, content experts' understanding of data strength and information management issues dramatically increases from the beginning of indicator development activities to the stage at which test data undergo assessment. Many content experts, for instance, who initially regarded diagnosis and coding as arcane and irrelevant to their professional lives later became quite adept and knowledgeable about these procedures and more, including identifying and addressing complex reliability and validity problems.

Fifth, methodology experts' understanding of clinical issues also increases. In the Joint Commission's experience, for example, methodology experts provided content experts with some important clinical insights they had gleaned from the field that had direct bearing on the data's reliability and validity; for example, the meaning of performing a Glasgow Coma Scale score for patients who had been pharmacologically paralyzed in the emergency department, or the confusion in the field about the meaning of "mechanical airway" (that is, whether it includes a bite block or esophageal obturator).

Summary Observations

Data interpreters must carefully weigh the strength of clinical performance data. Data that lack acceptable degrees of relevance, range, reliability, validity, variation, and control have the potential to impart irrelevant information (a waste of resources) or, worse, serious misinformation that can lead to poor decisions. The six attributes of strong clinical performance data are summarized below.

1. First, *relevance* is the degree to which clinical performance data relate to what organizations do—that is, functions or processes—and the relative importance of these functions or processes. Irrelevant data waste resources.

2. Second, addressing a wide *range* of health care processes and outcomes will give data users a complete portrait to accurately judge an organization's performance. This range will allow data users to invest improvement resources where they will do the most good and avoid causing (or failing to prevent) harm elsewhere in the organization.

3. Third, *data reliability* is the extent to which data results are consistent across repeated measurements of the same phenomenon by different measurers or at different times by the same measurers.

The phenomenon must not have changed in the interval between measurements. All data have a degree of unreliability. Nevertheless, an acceptable level of reliability should be present if data are to provide an accurate representation of the process or outcome undergoing measurement.

4. Fourth, *data validity* is the extent to which an indicator and its data measure only what they were intended to measure. The usefulness of data is directly related to the degree that they are valid in the eyes of users. Data reliability and validity are distinct, but interlinked, attributes that come in degrees. Unreliable data will almost always be invalid data. Reliable data, however, may not necessarily be valid data.

5. Fifth, *degree of variation* influences improvement opportunities. Wider variation in data usually signals more improvement opportunities, while narrower variation means fewer improvement opportunities. A large discrepancy between a data set's average value and what is generally the established and well-accepted (desired) average signals more improvement opportunities; a small discrepancy means fewer opportunities. Probably the greatest opportunity for improvement comes with data that show both wide variation with respect to their average *and* have an average that is displaced from the established average. The least opportunity for improvement comes with data that show narrow variation with respect to their average, which is *not* displaced from the established average.

6. Sixth, without *control* over the processes and outcomes undergoing measurement, improvement efforts can be both costly and futile.

References

1.   Brennan TA: The Health Security Act and improving the quality of care: Will the Clinton reforms help or hinder? In Jolt H (Ed): *U.S. Health Care In Transition: Reforming America's Health System Analysis, Reactions, Alternatives.* Philadelphia: Hanley & Belfus, 1994, pp 91–100.

2.   Kassirer JP: The use and abuse of practice profiles. *N Engl J Med* 330:634–636, 1994.

3.   Oberman L: Risk management strategy: Liability insurers stress practice guidelines. *American Medical News*, Sep 5, 1994, pp 1, 31.

4.   Winslow R: U.S. healthcare cuts costs, grows rapidly and irks some doctors. *Wall Street Journal*, Sep 6, 1994, pp A1, A8.

5.   Joint Commission on Accreditation of Healthcare Organizations: *Primer on Indicator Development and Application.* Oakbrook Terrace, IL: JCAHO, 1990, pp 26–27.

6.   Ibid, p 35.

7.   A clear look at cataracts. *Health Pages: A Consumer's Guide* pp 48–55, Summer/Fall, 1994.

8.   Prostate alert. *Health Pages: A Consumer Guide* pp 33–38, Winter, 1994.

9.   Provost P, Leddick S: How to take multiple measures to get a complete picture of organizational performance. *National Productivity Review* pp 477–489, Autumn 1993.

10.   Carmines EG, Zeller RA: *Reliability and Validity Assessment.* Sage University paper series on quantitative applications in the social sciences, 07-001. Beverly Hills, CA: Sage Publications, 1979, pp 37–51.

11.   Stanley JC: Reliability. In Thorndike RL (Ed): *Educational Measurement.* Washington, DC: American Council on Education, 1971, pp 356–442.

12.   Joint Commission on Accreditation of Healthcare Organizations: *The Measurement Mandate.* Oakbrook Terrace, IL: JCAHO, 1993, p 157.

13.   Carmines EG, Zeller RA: *Reliability and Validity Assessment.* Sage University paper series on quantitative applications in the social sciences, 07-001. Beverly Hills, CA: Sage Publications, 1979, pp 17–27.

14.   Joint Commission on Accreditation of Healthcare Organizations: *Lexikon: Dictionary of Health Care Terms, Organizations, and Acronyms for the Era of Reform.* Oakbrook Terrace, IL: JCAHO, 1994, p 237.

15. Cronbach LJ: Test validation. In Thorndike RL (Ed): *Educational Measurement.* Washington, DC: American Council on Education, 1971, pp 443–507.

16. Deming WE: *The New Economics for Industry, Government, Education.* Cambridge, MA: Massachusetts Institute of Technology Center for Advanced Engineering Study, 1993, pp 82, 130.

17. Ibid, p 193.

CHAPTER SIX

Summarizing
Clinical Performance Data

S trong clinical performance data can be readily transformed into accurate, useful performance summary information. *Summarizing data is the process of expressing unsorted raw data in a form that will permit, directly or by means of further calculations, conclusions to be drawn.* Specifically, it involves developing frequency distributions and calculating for these distributions measures of central tendency and data spread. Measures of central tendency and spread allow comparison between two or more frequency distributions, a topic addressed in Chapter Seven. When differences are observed between two distributions, interpreters are led to seek the reasons, or underlying factors, for the differences.

Clinical Performance Data and Their Frequency Distributions

Construction of a frequency distribution is often the first step in summarizing clinical performance data. In statistics, a *frequency distribution* (or, simply, distribution) is the complete summary of the frequencies of the values or categories of measurement made on a group of entities.[1] The distribution tells either how many or what proportion of the group was found to have each value (or each range of values) of all the possible values that the quantitative measure could have had. A *bell-shaped curve,* or *normal distribution,* is a familiar example of a distribution in which the greatest number of observations falls in the center with fewer and fewer observations falling evenly on either side of the average.

A distribution of indicator rates is constructed by first tabulating the unsorted rates for, say, a number of hospitals. Ideally, the number of groups should be limited to between 10 and 20.

For instance, consider constructing a frequency diagram for the indicator rates resulting from applying the following indicator:

> *Trauma patients with blood pressure, pulse rate, respiratory rate, and Glasgow Coma Scale score documented in the emergency department record on arrival and hourly until inpatient admission to the operating room or intensive care unit, death, or transfer to another care facility.**

The untabulated data for this indicator might look like Table 5 (see page 99): Hospital 1 has an indicator rate of 13%, Hospital 2 has an indicator rate of 60%, Hospital 3 has an indicator rate of 3%, and so on.

The rates can then be sorted into ten groups characterized by indicator rates of 0% to less than 10%, 10% to less than 20%, 20% to less than 30%, and so forth. The table would look like Table 6 (see page 100). For instance, of the 167 hospitals beta testing this particular Joint Commission trauma care indicator, 80 hospitals had rates that fell between 0% and 10%.

---

*This indicator was developed by the Joint Commission Trauma Care Task Force for Indicator Development. It was modified and improved, based on beta-testing results, and included in the IMSystem as the following two interrelated indicators (Indicators 21A and 21B):

> *Trauma patients with blood pressure, pulse, and respiration documented on arrival and at least hourly for three hours, or until emergency department disposition, whichever is earlier; and*
> *Trauma patients with selected intracranial injuries with Glasgow Coma Scale score documented on arrival and at least hourly for three hours, or until emergency department disposition, whichever is earlier.*

TABLE 5 Sample of Unsorted Indicator Data for Beta Indicator TR-2*

Hospital Identity	TR-2 Indicator Rate for Specified Time Period
Hospital 1	13%
Hospital 2	60%
Hospital 3	3%
Hospital 4	2%
Hospital 5	11%
Hospital 6	6%
Hospital 7	4%
Hospital 8	7%
and so on	

*TR-2: Trauma patients with blood pressure, pulse, respirations, and Glasgow Coma Scale score documented in the emergency department record on arrival and hourly until inpatient admission to the operating room or intensive care unit, death, or transfer to another care facility.

The final step in constructing a distribution is to use the tabulated data to create a diagram that brings out the main features of the data. One expert notes that a frequency diagram "often assists the intelligence to grasp the meaning of a series of numbers by means of the eye."[2] The distribution for the clinical performance data that were tabulated in Table 6 is shown graphically in Figure 9 (see page 101) as a histogram. Note that the data are not normally distributed; rather, they are skewed to the right.

A second example of a frequency distribution uses indicator rates resulting from applying the following indicator:

Trauma patients undergoing laparotomy for wounds penetrating the abdominal wall.[†]

---

† This indicator was developed by the Joint Commission Trauma Care Task Force for Indicator Development but was not recommended for inclusion in the IMSystem.

TABLE 6 Table of Sorted Hospital Indicator Rates for Beta Indicator TR-2

Indicator Rate	Number of Hospitals
0% to less than 10%	80
10% to less than 20%	15
20% to less than 30%	17
30% to less than 40%	14
40% to less than 50%	8
50% to less than 60%	12
60% to less than 70%	8
70% to less than 80%	6
80% to less than 90%	6
90% to 100%	1
Total number of beta hospitals contributing data for this indicator:	167

Table 7. Sample of Unsorted Indicator Data for Indicator TR-8*

Hospital Identity	Indicator Rate for Specified Time Period
Hospital 1	5%
Hospital 2	90%
Hospital 3	52%
Hospital 4	2%
Hospital 5	66%
Hospital 6	92%
Hospital 7	71%
Hospital 8	58%
and so forth	

* TR-8:Trauma patients undergoing laparotomy for wounds penetrating the abdominal wall.

FIGURE 9 Frequency Distribution for Beta Hospital Indicator Rates for Indicator TR-2

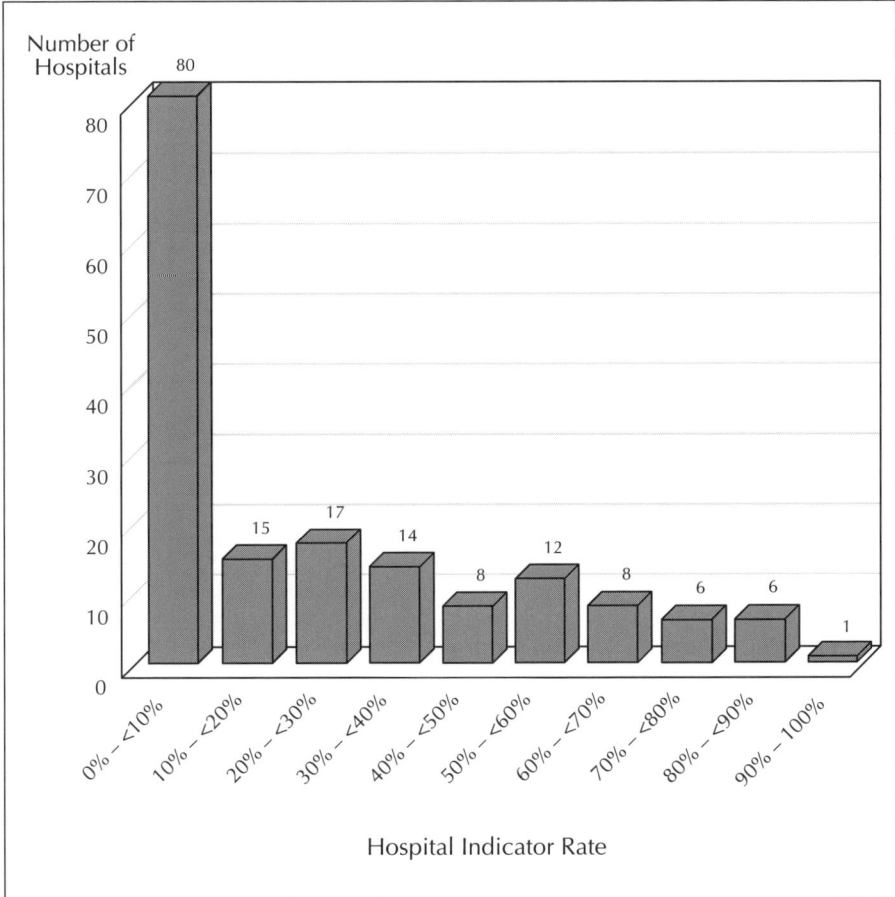

This histogram shows how many hospitals were in each percentage group for the TR-2 indicator (documenting hourly vital signs, including Glasgow Coma Scale score, for trauma patients). Note that 80 of 167 hospitals had indicator rates below 10%.

The untabulated data for this indicator are in Table 7 (see page 100): Hospital 1 has an indicator rate of 5%, Hospital 2 has an indicator rate of 90%, Hospital 3 has an indicator rate of 52%, and so forth. The sorted, tabulated data are in Table 8 (see page 102). The frequency distribution of these data is presented in Figure 10 (see page 103) as a histogram.

TABLE 8 Sorted Hospital Indicator Rates for Indicator TR-8

Indicator Rate	Number of Hospitals
0% to less than 10%	19
10% to less than 20%	1
20% to less than 30%	1
30% to less than 40%	11
40% to less than 50%	7
50% to less than 60%	23
60% to less than 70%	7
70% to less than 80%	8
80% to less than 90%	2
90% to 100%	21
Total number of beta hospitals contributing data for this indicator:	100

A third example of a frequency distribution uses indicator rates resulting from applying the following indicator:

> *Trauma patients with prehospital emergency medical services scene times of greater than 20 minutes.*[*]

The frequency distribution of these indicator data is shown in Figure 11 (see page 104).

However, this same indicator could generate a different frequency distribution. Prehospital scene times could be sorted into groups characterized by the mean (average) number of minutes spent at trauma scenes by prehospital emergency medical services personnel, as reported by the hospitals to which the patients were eventually transported. A distribution of these time data graphed as a frequency diagram would look like Figure 12 (see page 105).

---

[*] This indicator was developed by the Joint Commission Trauma Care Task Force for Indicator Development but was not recommended for inclusion in the IMSystem.

FIGURE 10 Frequency Distribution for Beta Hospital Indicator Rates for Indicator TR-8

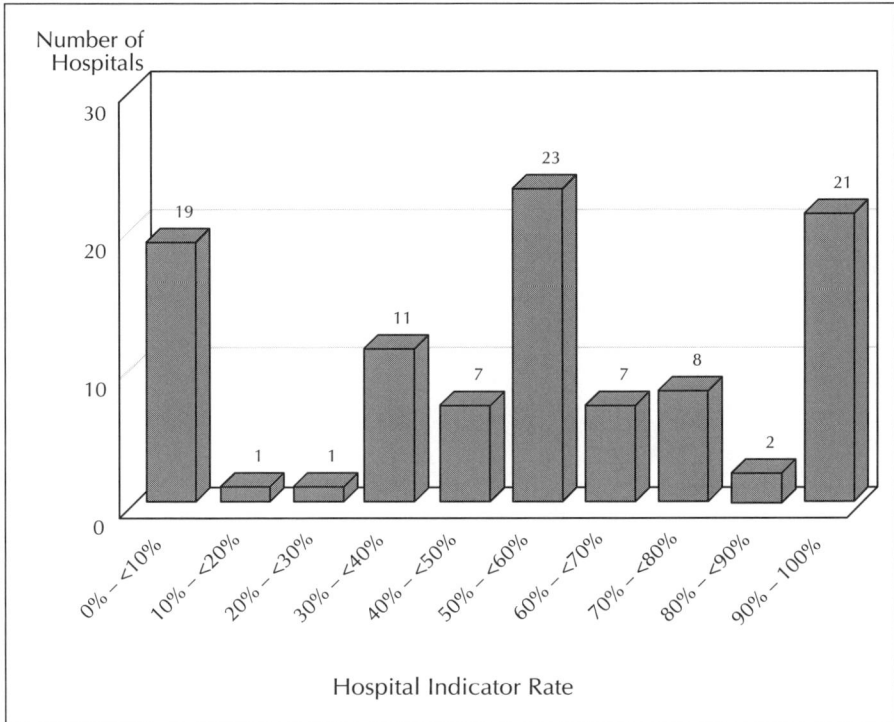

This histogram shows the number and corresponding percentage group of hospitals for indicator TR-8 (trauma patients undergoing laparotomy for wounds penetrating the abdominal wall).

Important Characteristics of Distributions of Clinical Performance Data

The next step after putting a series of observations in the form of a frequency distribution is to calculate certain important values that describe the distribution's characteristics. These values—measures of central tendency and spread—enable data interpreters to make comparisons between one set of clinical performance data and another.

For instance, suppose that a hospital's mean indicator rate for some process of care is 20% one year and 80% the next year. Or consider that the hospital's mean indicator rate for some process is 20% and the mean indicator rate for all peer hospitals is 60%. In

FIGURE 11 Frequency Distribution for Beta Hospital Indicator Rates for Indicator TR-1

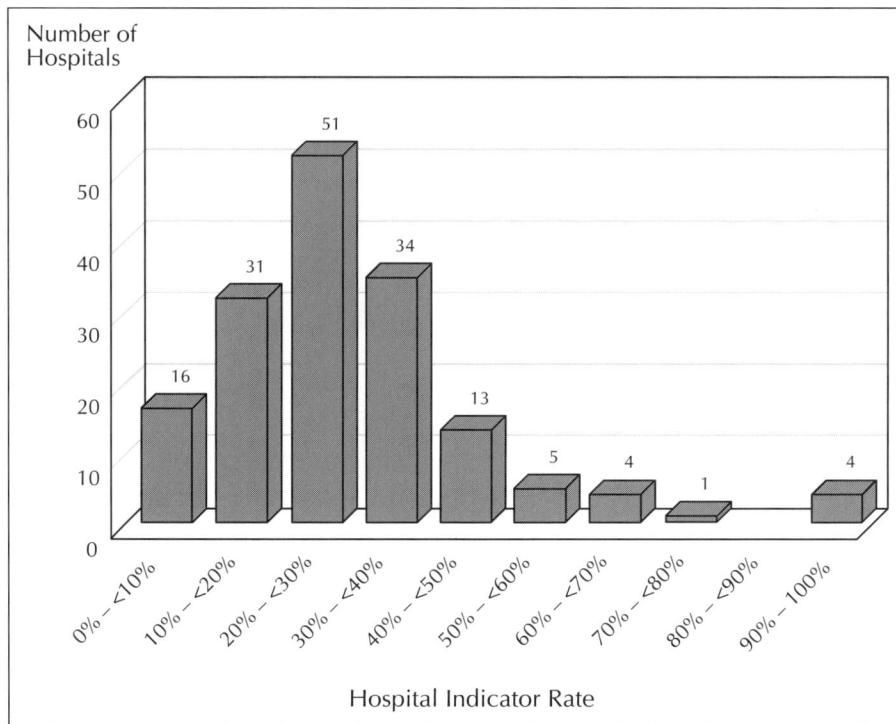

This histogram shows the number of hospitals in each percentage group for indicator TR-1 (trauma patients with emergency medical services scene times greater than 20 minutes).

both instances, the distribution of the hospital's data differs in its comparative position: 20% versus 80%, and 20% versus 60%. As will be discussed in Chapter Seven, this observed difference should lead interpreters to seek out underlying factors that explain the difference. The intent of identifying the factors is to remedy the discrepancy, or decrease the observed variation. *It is extremely important to remember that the hospital with an outlier value for a given process or outcome undergoing measurement may actually be providing the most desired level of care.* In such a case, decreasing observed variation may well involve moving other hospitals' values (and practices resulting in the values) toward that of the outlier hospital.

FIGURE 12 Frequency Distribution for Beta Hospital Mean Scene Time (in Minutes) for Indicator TR-1

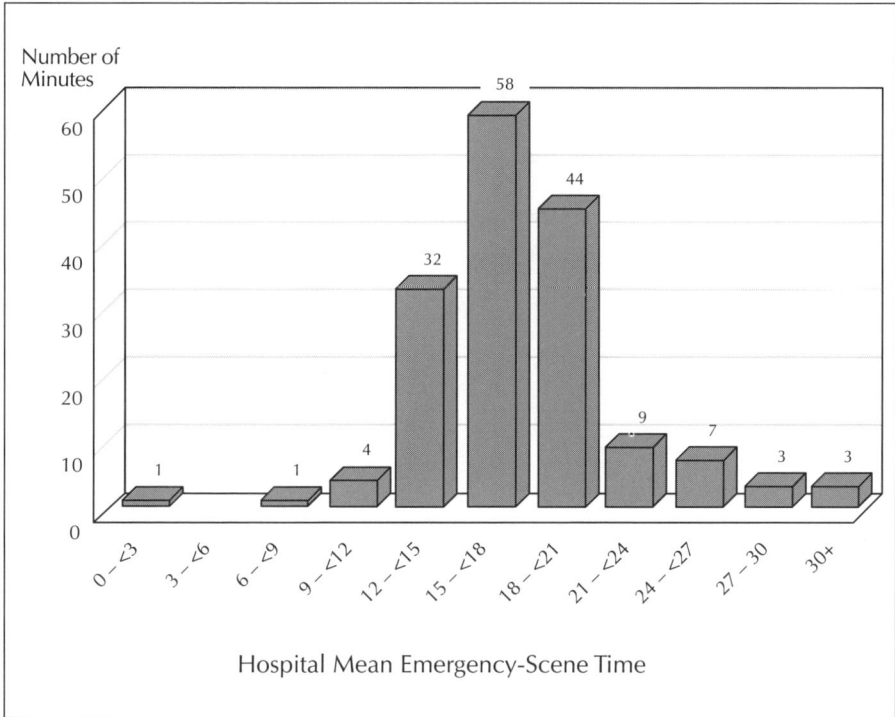

This histogram shows the average number of minutes emergency medical services personnel spent at trauma scenes and the number of hospitals in each average range.

Measures of Central Tendency for Clinical Performance Data Distributions

The median, mean, and mode are three measures of central tendency for a given data set's frequency distribution (see Table 9, page 106).

Median. The median of a data set's distribution is the middle number when the measurements are arranged sequentially from smallest to largest or from largest to smallest. Therefore, the median is the most valid measure of central tendency whenever a distribution is skewed.[3]

For instance, a group of hospitals may have indicator rates of between 10% and 15% for a particular outcome. The median will not

TABLE 9 Measures of Central Tendency

Median: The middle value of a set of clinical performance data

Mean: The average value of a set of clinical performance data

Mode: The most common value of a set of clinical performance data

be altered much by the addition of two more hospitals with indicator rates between 90% and 95%. These two hospitals represent cases lying above the middle point, but how much above is immaterial.

The median is often used in conjunction with the interquartile range, which is described on page 112.

Mean. The mean of a data set's distribution specifies the data set's arithmetic average—that is, the sum of all the measurements divided by the total number of measurements in the data set.

The mean is best used as a measure of central tendency when the distribution of data is balanced and when data are evenly distributed around a single value, as in a normal, bell-shaped curve. However, the mean, in contrast to the median, may be affected by large outlying measurements, such as in skewed, or asymmetric, distributions. A median will be relatively unaffected by large outlying measurements.[4]

Again, in a group of hospitals with indicator rates between 10% and 15% for a certain outcome, the *median* will not be altered much by the addition of two more hospitals with indicator rates between 90% and 95%, but the *mean* may be increased. In such a case, the mean is a less satisfactory measure of the distribution's central location.

Mode. The mode of a data set's distribution is the value that occurs most often.[5]

In normally distributed clinical performance data, the mean and median (also the mode) are identical (see Figure 13A, page 108). When the mean is greater than the median, the distribution will be right-skewed (see Figure 13B). When the mean is less than the median, the distribution will be left-skewed (see Figure 13C).

Measures of Dispersion for Clinical Performance Data Distributions

By itself, the data set's central location is of limited value because it provides no information about the dispersion (also called spread, scatter, or variability) of measurements. For example, a group of hospitals has a mean indicator rate of 50% for a care process with an established indicator rate of 50%. Without knowledge of the data set's dispersion, one might conclude that the group of hospitals performed well on this particular care process. However, the hospitals' rates ranged between 0% and 100%, with a calculated mean of 50%. The data suddenly become more interesting. Opportunities to improve care may be abundant among the hospitals whose rates are dispersed far from the group's mean. These opportunities would have been missed if just the data set's mean had been used for interpretation.

There are three important measures of dispersion: the *range,* the *standard deviation,* and the *interquartile range* (see Table 10, page 109). As described below, the interquartile range is generally more useful in summarizing and comparing clinical performance data than the range and standard deviation.

Range. The range is the distance between the lowest and highest values in a data set. It is calculated by subtracting the lowest value in the data set from the highest value in that same set. Its usefulness as a measure of dispersion is limited because it is based on only the two extreme values in a data set and ignores the distribution of all the values within those limits. Two data sets may have identical ranges but very different-looking variabilities because the data points are configured differently between the mean and the outlying values (see Figure 14, page 110).

FIGURE 13 Relationship of the Mean, Median, and Mode to a Distribution's Skew

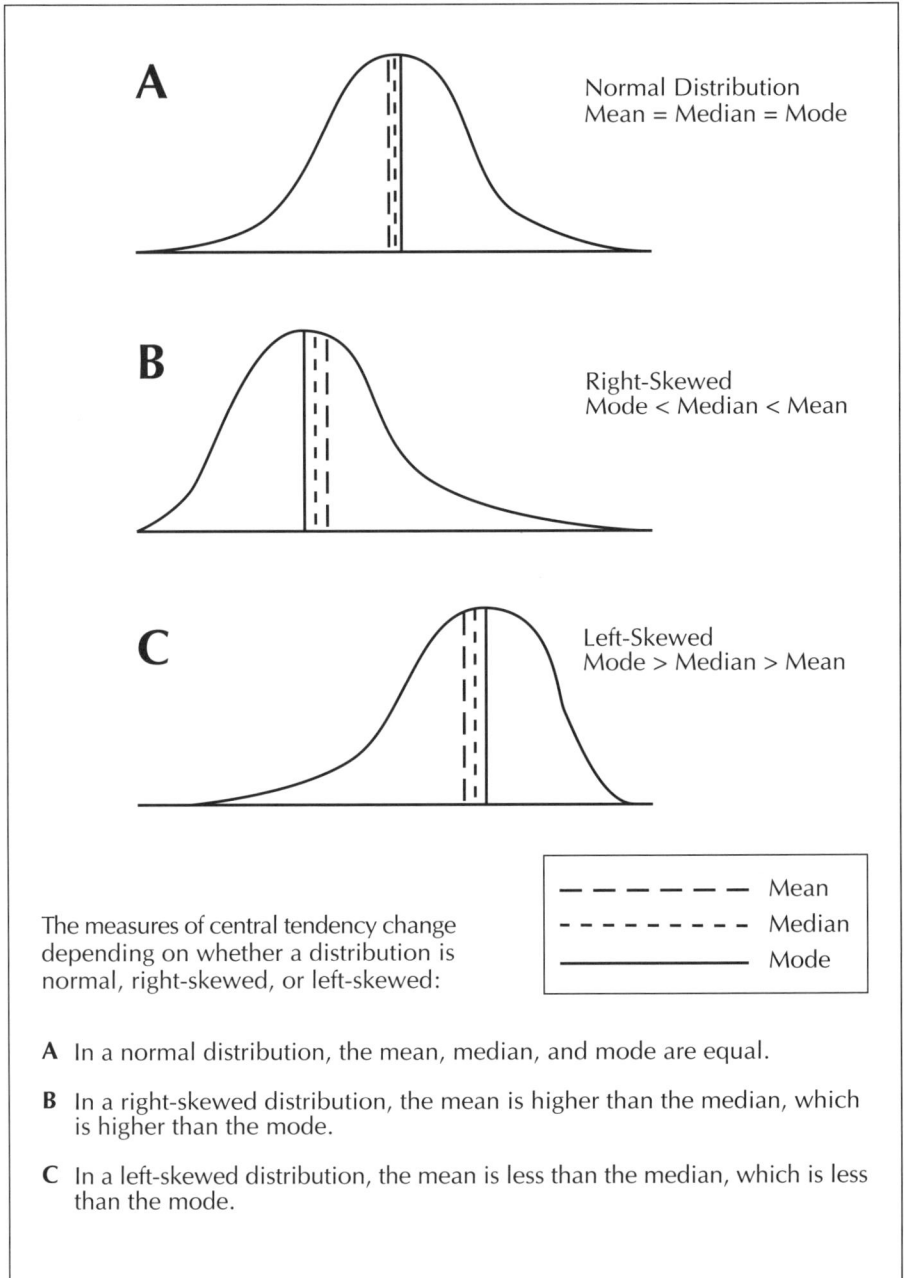

A — Normal Distribution
Mean = Median = Mode

B — Right-Skewed
Mode < Median < Mean

C — Left-Skewed
Mode > Median > Mean

The measures of central tendency change depending on whether a distribution is normal, right-skewed, or left-skewed:

– – – – – – Mean
- - - - - - - - Median
———— Mode

A In a normal distribution, the mean, median, and mode are equal.

B In a right-skewed distribution, the mean is higher than the median, which is higher than the mode.

C In a left-skewed distribution, the mean is less than the median, which is less than the mode.

The figure above illustrates measures of central tendency change depending on whether a distribution is normal, right-skewed, or left-skewed.

TABLE 10 Measures of Dispersion

Range:	The difference between the lowest and highest values in a set of clinical performance data
Standard Deviation:	The square root of the variance
Interquartile Range:	The range covered by the middle 50% of the values in a set of clinical performance data

Standard deviation. The standard deviation is another measure of a distribution's spread. It is equal to the square root of the mean of all the squares of the deviations from the mean.[6] The standard deviation is calculated for a data set in the following way.

For a data set that contains five indicator rates of 10%, 20%, 40%, 70%, and 90%, the arithmetic mean calculates to 46%. The deviation from this mean of 46% can be calculated for each of the five measurements in the following manner:

Deviation from the mean of 46%:

Indicator Mean		Indicator Rate		Indicator Deviation	Square of Deviation
46	–	10	=	36	1,296
46	–	20	=	26	676
46	–	40	=	6	36
46	–	70	=	–24	576
46	–	90	=	–44	1,936

Then the squares are added and the sum is divided by 5 (the number of measurements in the data set):

$$\frac{1{,}296 + 676 + 36 + 576 + 1{,}936}{5} = \frac{4{,}520}{5} = 904$$

The quotient, 904, is called the *variance.* The standard deviation is

FIGURE 14 Two Data Sets with Identical Ranges and Different Variabilities

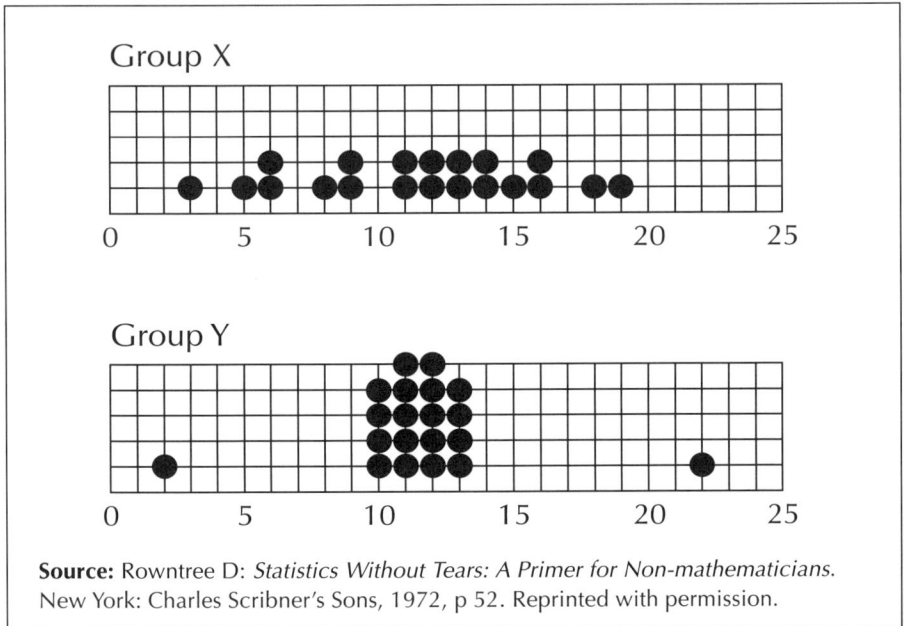

Source: Rowntree D: *Statistics Without Tears: A Primer for Non-mathematicians.* New York: Charles Scribner's Sons, 1972, p 52. Reprinted with permission.

In this figure, Group X and Group Y have the same range of values (0–25), but Group Y's distribution is clustered around the mean.

the square root of the variance. The square root of 904 is 30.07, so the standard deviation for this data set is 30.07.

The standard deviation's relationship to the values falling within a normal curve is constant. The standard deviation divides a bell-shaped distribution into standard-sized slices, and each slice contains a known percentage of the total values in the data set.[7] Sixty-eight percent of the values in a normal distribution will fall within one standard deviation either side of the mean, 95% of the values will lie within about two (actually, 1.96) standard deviations either side of the mean, and 99.7% of the values in a data set will lie within three standard deviations either side of the mean (see Figure 15, page 111). A large standard deviation shows that the distribution is widely spread out from the mean, while a small standard deviation shows that it lies closely concentrated about the mean with little variability between one value and another (see

FIGURE 15 Standard Deviation and Areas Under a Normal Curve

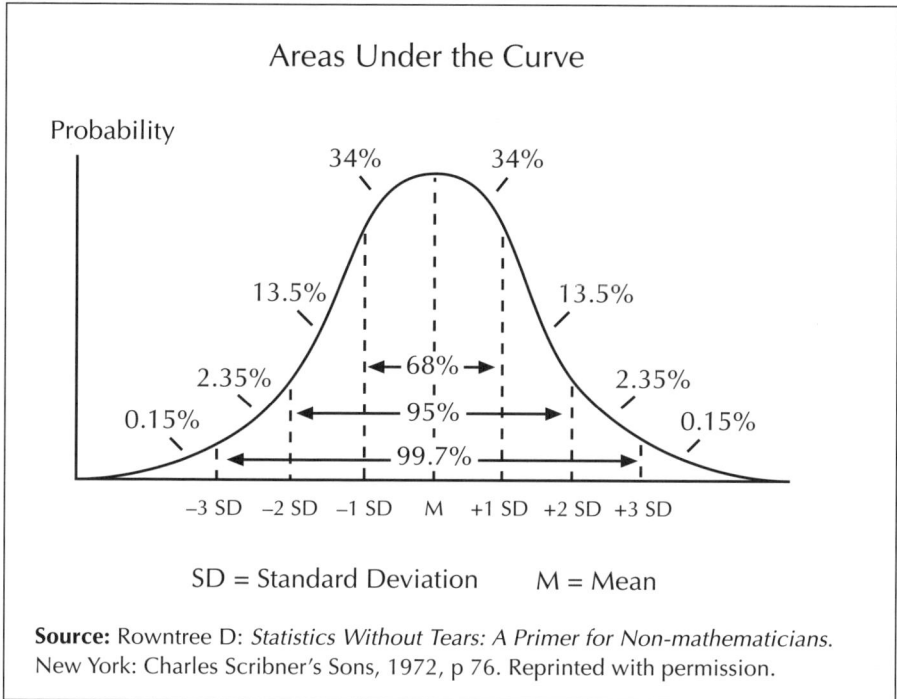

Areas Under the Curve

Probability

34%   34%

13.5%   13.5%

2.35% ←68%→ 2.35%

0.15% ←95%→ 0.15%

←99.7%→

–3 SD –2 SD –1 SD M +1 SD +2 SD +3 SD

SD = Standard Deviation   M = Mean

Source: Rowntree D: *Statistics Without Tears: A Primer for Non-mathematicians.* New York: Charles Scribner's Sons, 1972, p 76. Reprinted with permission.

The standard deviation divides a normal curve into segments, each segment containing a known percentage of the total values in the data set. Sixty-eight percent of the values in a normal distribution will fall within one standard deviation either side of the mean, 95% within two standard deviations, and 99.7% within three standard deviations.

Figure 8A [large standard deviation] and 8B [small standard deviation] in Chapter Five).

The standard deviation has two main purposes. First, it provides a convenient way of summarizing the difference in distributions by measuring the variability of each distribution in a single number (statistic). Second, as will be discussed in Chapter Seven, the standard deviation enables data interpreters to test whether the differences in range (variability) observed between two distributions (say, a hospital's distribution and the distribution of all similar hospitals for a given indicator over a specified period of time) are more than would be likely to have arisen by chance alone (that is, is the difference significant?).[8]

The standard deviation tool has one major limitation. Standard deviations are useful in describing the range for curves that are normal distributions but most data sets fall under *nonnormal*, rather than normal, distributions. *The standard deviation is meaningless in non-normally distributed data* because the proportions under the curve are not reasonably close to those predicted by the normal curve. (For example, far more or less than 68% of the data set's values may fall within one standard deviation above and below the mean.) When data are not normally distributed, the most meaningful measure of dispersion is the interquartile range.

Interquartile range. Any frequency distribution can be divided into equal, ordered subgroups called *quantiles*. Centile, decile, quintile, and tercile are quantiles for distributions divided into hundredths, tenths, fifths, and thirds, respectively.

Four *quartiles* divide a distribution into four equal parts. A quartile's boundary is at the 25th, 50th, or 75th percentiles of such a distribution. The first quartile (Q1) is the point below which 25% of the values in the data set lie. The second quartile (Q2) falls at the distribution's median. The third quartile (Q3) is the point below which 75% of the values lie.

Interquartile range is a measure of dispersion around the median of a distribution (see Figure 16, page 113). To calculate interquartile range, all values in the data set must first be arranged in increasing order. Then the distribution is divided into equal subgroups, meaning that 25% of the values will lie between the minimum value and Q1, 25% of the values between Q1 and Q2, 25% of the values between Q2 and Q3, and 25% of the values between Q3 and the maximum value of the data set. The interquartile range is the range in values between Q1 (25% of the observations) and Q3 (75% of the observations).

How important is the interquartile range as a tool in describing

FIGURE 16 Interquartile Range: A Measure of Dispersion Around the Median of a Distribution

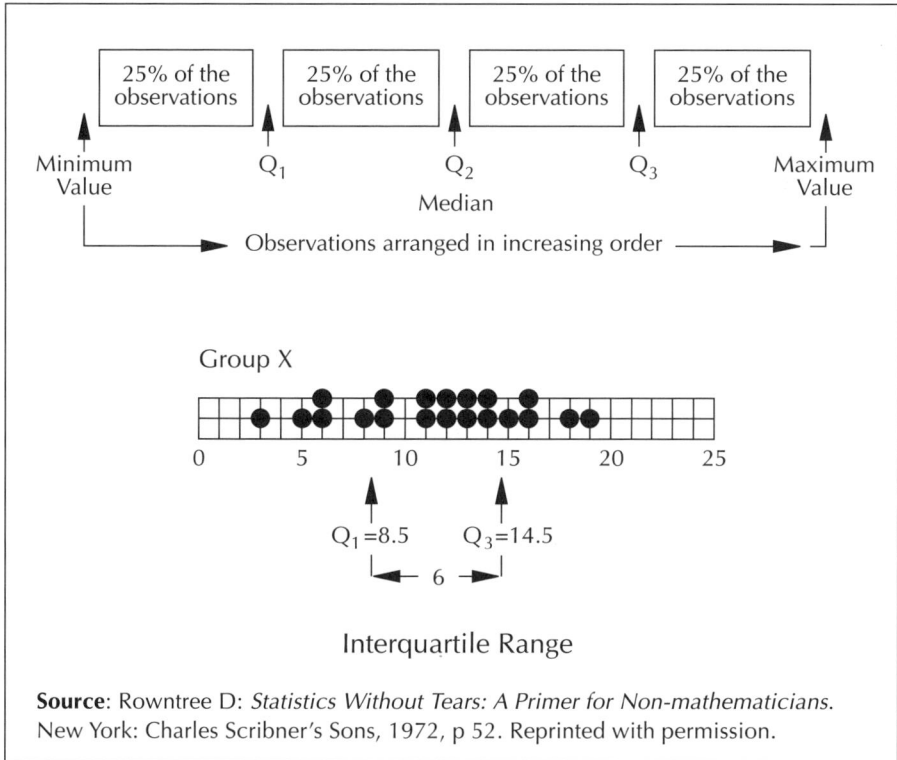

Source: Rowntree D: *Statistics Without Tears: A Primer for Non-mathematicians.* New York: Charles Scribner's Sons, 1972, p 52. Reprinted with permission.

After dividing the data's distribution into four equal subgroups (Q=quartile), the interquartile range will encompass values between 25% and 75% of the observations.

the dispersion of a data set? To demonstrate its importance, consider the following indicator:

> *Comatose patients discharged from the emergency department prior to the establishment of a mechanical airway.**

Joint Commission beta test site data (seven calendar quarters of data collected from 103 test site hospitals) showed that the *mean*

---

* This indicator was developed by the Joint Commission Trauma Care Task Force for Indicator Development and was selected in a revised form for inclusion in the IMSystem.

indicator rate for this process of care was approximately 20%. This means that for these 103 hospitals, comatose trauma patients were discharged from the emergency department before a mechanical airway was established (that is, endotracheal intubation or cricothyrotomy) an average of 20% of the time (one in five comatose patients did not have a mechanical airway established before discharge from the emergency department). However, the *standard deviation* for the distribution was approximately 26%.

The astute reader may ask how a standard deviation can be greater than the mean for this distribution. The answer is, it can't if the distribution is normal. A standard deviation greater than the mean implies the existence of negative indicator rates for this process of care, which is impossible. *A major clue that a distribution is* not *normally distributed is when the standard deviation is equal to or greater than half the mean (and when negative numbers are not possible).*

The median and interquartile range are better suited for non-normal distributions because they are less sensitive to outlying values. The *median* indicator rate for the distribution of comatose patients already described was 11%, meaning that half the hospitals had indicator rates greater than 11% and half had indicator rates less than 11%. The *interquartile range* (Q1–Q3) for the distribution was 0% to 33%, meaning that the middle 50% of the hospitals had indicator rates in the range of 0% to 33%. Since the minimum value for the data set was also 0%, one can also say that 75% of the hospitals had indicator rates less than 33%.

Sampling Distributions

Many of the statistical techniques previously described depend on the existence of a normal distribution. But there are many cases for which a population cannot be assumed to be normal in distribution. For example, some of the Joint Commission's beta-testing indicator data are not normally distributed because the indicators used in beta testing generated attribute (discrete variable) data. As previously described in Chapter Four, the type of data—attribute versus continuous variable data—is an important characteristic of clinical performance data.

Attribute data have only two possible values: indicator occurrence or nonoccurrence. For instance, in any indicator that measures patient mortality, the patient either dies or survives. Indicator occurrences exist when the conditions specified in indicator statements are met.

The idea of a normal distribution is inappropriate to attribute data.[9] Nevertheless, the distributions of certain statistics calculated for attribute data *do* follow certain known probability models, including normal distributions. In analytic studies, these distributions are called *sampling distributions of statistics.*

One sampling distribution is the *mean of the sample means.* Each sample of attribute data will have its own mean. These means can be compared in size from smallest to largest, and the amount of means in each size can also be determined. The result is a frequency distribution of the sample means, which will have its own mean called the mean of the sample means. *The distribution's shape for the mean of the sample means will be normal, even when the population is not normally distributed.*

This observation is critical to constructing control charts for attribute data, described fully in Chapter Seven. If a large enough number of samples is gathered, the mean of the sample means will approach the population mean, which is the same as the overall indicator rate. The mean of the sample means is also the center line of a control chart and the mean for the process or outcome undergoing analysis.

Another sampling distribution is the *distribution of sample means.* The standard deviation of a sampling distribution is called the *standard error.* This distinguishes it from the standard deviation of a sample or of the population. The standard error enables interpreters to calculate the chances that a particular sample mean will be much larger or smaller than the population mean.[10] The standard error is needed for control charts because their upper and lower control limits are based on this statistic. The standard error is discussed further in Chapter Seven.

In brief, sampling distributions are important because they enable interpreters to construct control charts that ascertain the stability of a process and identify opportunities for improvement. Sampling distributions enable interpreters to make inferences from samples or subgroups as a basis for taking action on the population under study.

One Approach to Summarizing Clinical Performance Data

One approach to summarizing clinical performance data was used by the Joint Commission for beta indicator data that were transmitted from beta-testing hospitals to the Joint Commission's performance database. Each indicator's data were summarized for all beta-testing hospitals (Total Database Description) and for individual hospitals (Hospital Level Description). The following indicator (TR-1) is used as an example for the following descriptions:

> *Trauma patients with prehospital emergency medical services scene times of greater than 20 minutes.**

Total Database Description. The analysis of the total database was divided into eight sections (see Table 11, page 117).

1. The first section is the number of cases with insufficient information to determine whether the case was a member of the denominator population. This group of cases are referred to as Category I cases. When a crucial data element was missing from a hospital's transmission to the Joint Commission database, the case was isolated from the remaining cases. The computer software kept track of these cases as Category I cases. This group of cases provides hospitals with valuable information concerning opportunities to improve management of information.

---

* This indicator was developed by the Joint Commission Trauma Care Task Force for Indicator Development but was not recommended for inclusion in the IMSystem.

TABLE 11 Summary Data for Indicator TR-1*

Total Database Description	TR-1
1. Insufficient information to determine denominator status	4,801
2. Not part of the indicator population	14,682
3. Insufficient information to determine numerator status	20,741
4. Indicator denominator, but not numerator	21,776
5. Indicator numerator, but not denominator	7,372
6. Overall indicator rate = V ÷ (IV+V)	25.3%
7. Percentage of trauma population not eligible for indicator population = II ÷ (I+II+III+IV+V)	21.2%
8. Percentage of potential numerator or denominator cases lost due to missing data = (I+III) ÷ (I+III+IV+V)	46.7%
Hospital Level Description	
1. Number of hospitals reporting denominator cases for this indicator	158
2. Median hospital indicator rate	25.4
3. Interquartile range indicator rate	(17.3, 34.7)
4. Median hospital denominator cases	94
5. Interquartile range for denominator cases	(34, 234)
6. Median hospital percentage not eligible	22.6%
7. Interquartile range for percentage not eligible	(13.5, 32.3)
8. Median hospital percentage missing	39.7%
9. Interquartile range for percentage missing	(19.0, 63.8)

* Trauma patients with prehospital emergency medical services scene times of greater than 20 minutes.

Source: Joint Commission beta database

According to beta data produced by indicator TR-1, the number of cases with insufficient information to determine whether the case was a member of the denominator population was 4,801. Each Category I case for this indicator was missing the data element *mode of transportation of patients from the scene of injury* (for example, by ambulance, helicopter, fixed wing, public safety vehicle, private vehicle, walk-in). Without knowing this initial data element, it was impossible to determine whether the case was part of the denominator population, which was defined as the number of trauma patients transported by emergency medical services (EMS).

2. The second section is the number of cases with sufficient information to determine whether the case was a member of the denominator population but they were not determined to be not part of the denominator population. This group of cases is referred to as Category II cases. For these cases, sufficient crucial data elements had been successfully transmitted by beta-testing hospitals to the Joint Commission database. The determination could thus be made that the case *did not belong* to the denominator population. These Category II cases, tracked by computer software, were isolated from the remaining cases.

According to beta data generated by TR-1, the number of cases with sufficient information to determine that the case was *not* a member of the denominator population was 14,682. This means that of the 69,372 cases of trauma patients in the database, 14,682 did not meet the explicit requirements for indicator TR-1, which were patient arrival at the hospital by ambulance, helicopter, or fixed-wing aircraft (emergency medical services).

3. The third section is the number of cases with insufficient information to determine whether the case belonged in the numerator population. This group of cases is referred to as Category III cases. This means that certain other data elements were missing from hospitals' transmissions to the Joint Commission database. These Category III cases were isolated from the remaining cases of the numerator population and tracked by the computer.

Beta data produced by indicator TR-1 showed that the number of cases with insufficient information to determine whether the case was a member of the numerator population was 20,741. Of these 20,741 cases, the ambulance run report was not present (14,697 cases), the EMS scene arrival date and time were missing from the run report (5,274 cases), or the EMS scene departure date and time were missing from the run report (770 cases). Each of these data elements was critical to determining whether a case was part of the numerator population.

4. The fourth section is the number of cases that belong to the indicator denominator population, but not including those in the indicator numerator. This group of cases is referred to as Category IV cases. This means that all required data elements had been successfully transmitted by beta hospitals to the Joint Commission database. The determination could thus be made that the case *did belong* to the denominator population. These cases, tracked as Category IV by the computer, made up the denominator of indicator rates.

According to beta data produced by indicator TR-1, the number of cases with sufficient information to determine that the case was a member of the denominator population was 21,776. This means that 21,776 trauma patients were transported by EMS and all additional necessary data elements were available to determine whether EMS scene time was greater than 20 minutes.

5. The fifth section is the number of cases that belong to the indicator numerator population, but not the denominator population (Category V). This means that all required data elements had been successfully transmitted by beta hospitals to the Joint Commission database. The determination could thus be made that the case *did belong* to the numerator population. These cases made up the numerator of indicator rates. The computer software kept track of them as Category V cases.

Beta data generated by indicator TR-1 showed that the number of cases for which there was sufficient information to determine that the case was a member of the numerator population was 7,372. This means that 7,372 of 21,776 trauma patients who were transported by EMS to the hospital had EMS scene times of greater than 20 minutes.

6. The sixth section is the overall indicator rate (V ÷ [IV + V]) for the database. This calculation is performed by dividing the number of cases in the numerator by the number of cases in the denominator plus the number of cases in the numerator. For indicator TR-1, V ÷ (IV + V) is calculated as follows:

$$\frac{7{,}372}{21{,}776 + 7{,}372} = \frac{7{,}372}{29{,}148} = 25.3\%$$

Thus, 25.3% of trauma patients transported by EMS had scene times longer than 20 minutes. This 25.3% rate is the database's mean indicator rate for TR-1 at a given point in time.

7. The seventh section is the percent of the trauma population in the database that is not eligible for the indicator population (II ÷ [I + II + III + IV + V]). This formula measures how many trauma cases were ineligible for the indicator population simply because they did not meet requirements for the indicator, not because of problems with missing data. For indicator TR-1 beta data, of the 69,372 cases of trauma patients in the database, 14,682 did not meet the explicit requirements for the indicator—that is, 21.2% of trauma patients in this database arrived at the hospital emergency departments by means *other than* ambulance, helicopter, or fixed-wing aircraft.

8. The eighth section is the percent of potential numerator or denominator cases lost due to missing data ([I + III] ÷ [I + III + IV + V]). This formula measures how many cases are lost to interpretation because of missing data. It is an important measure because opportunities to improve care are often related to management of information, including documentation of that care. Opportunities to improve a process of care may be severely limited until documentation of the care can first be improved. For indicator TR-1, almost half (46.7%) of all potential cases were lost because of missing data.

__Hospital Level Description.__ The analysis of the database for
individual hospitals was divided into nine sections (see Table 11,
page 117).

1. The first section is the number of hospitals reporting denominator cases for a specified indicator. This number refers to the
number of test site hospitals that contributed denominator (indicator
population) cases to the database for a specified indicator. For the
indicator TR-1, 158 test site hospitals reported denominator cases.

The number varies by indicator depending in part on whether
the hospital cared for one or more patients with the occurrence
measured by the indicator during a specified time period. If, for
instance, a hospital did not offer a specified type of procedure, such
as coronary artery bypass graft surgery, it would not be able to
collect and transmit any cases involving coronary artery bypass graft
surgery to the Joint Commission database. The number of hospitals
for that indicator would be one less than the total number of test
site hospitals agreeing to test the set of, in this case, cardiovascular
indicators.

2. The second section is the median hospital indicator rate,
which is the middle number of an indicator's distribution when the
rates are arranged sequentially from smallest to largest or from
largest to smallest. As previously noted, the median is the most valid
measure of central tendency whenever a distribution is skewed, and
is often used in conjunction with the interquartile range. The test
sites' indicator distributions tended to be asymmetric for many of the
Joint Commission indicators. For indicator TR-1, the median and
mean happened to be very close (25.4% versus 25.3%). The actual
distribution for TR-1 hospital indicator rates is portrayed in Figure
11 on page 104.

3. The third section is the interquartile range indicator rate. The
interquartile range, as previously described, is a measure of the dispersion around a distribution's median (see Figure 16, page 113). For the
beta data generated by indicator TR-1, the interquartile range is 17.3%
to 34.7% around a median of 25.4. This means that 50% of the hospital

indicator rates lie between 17.3% and 34.7%. Since we know that the third quartile is the point below which 75% of the values lie, we can say that 75% of hospital indicator rates for TR-1 lie below 34.7%.

4. The fourth section is the median hospital denominator cases, which is the middle number of the hospitals' distribution according to their number of denominator cases, when the number of denominator cases per hospital is arranged sequentially from smallest to largest or from largest to smallest.

According to beta data produced by indicator TR-1, the median for hospital denominator cases was 94, meaning that 94 cases relating to TR-1 represented the middle number of a distribution of test site hospitals arranged from lowest to highest, according to the number of denominator cases that they transmitted to the Joint Commission during a specified time period.

The median for hospital denominator cases was used as an important measure of the relevance (or significance) of an indicator. Indicators with a very small median number of cases per hospital (say 1 or 2 per time period) would probably be less useful to hospitals and the Joint Commission because the occurrences being measured happened so rarely. By contrast, indicators with a large median number of cases per hospital would probably be more useful to hospitals and the Joint Commission because the occurrence being measured happened more frequently.

5. The fifth section is interquartile range for hospital denominator cases. The interquartile range for indicator TR-1 is 34–234. This means that 50% of the hospitals transmitted between 34 cases and 234 cases during the time period of interest. Remembering that the third quartile is the point below which 75% of the values lie, we can say that 75% of hospitals transmitted fewer than 234 denominator cases for TR-1 during the time period of interest.

6. The sixth section is median hospital percent not eligible. This measure is related to the seventh section of the Total Database Description on page 120. Instead of describing the mean, however, which was described in the Total Database Description, this measure

describes the median for the distribution. For indicator TR-1, the median hospital percent not eligible was 22.6% (compared to a mean of 21.2%). Thus, the distribution *should* be slightly left-skewed because the mean is less than the median (see Figure 13C, page 108).

7. The seventh section is interquartile range for percent not eligible. According to beta data produced by indicator TR-1, the interquartile range for percent not eligible is 13.5% to 32.3%. This means that for 75% of beta-testing hospitals, 32.3% of their cases transmitted to the Joint Commission were ineligible for the TR-1 indicator population simply because these cases did not meet requirements for the indicator. The cases had no problems with missing data. They were relevant to other trauma indicators.

8. The eighth section is median hospital percent missing. This is closely related to the eighth section of Total Database Description previously described except that the median, rather than the mean, is addressed. For indicator TR-1 beta data, the median hospital was losing 39.7% of cases potentially relevant to interpretation because of missing data. Compared to the previously reported mean of 46.7%, we can predict from the median that the distribution for median hospital percent missing is right-skewed: the mean is larger than the median (see Figure 13B, page 108).

9. The ninth section is interquartile range for hospital percent missing, which is based on the distribution described in the previous section. The interquartile range for indicator TR-1 is 19.0% to 63.8%, meaning that 75% of test site hospitals were losing 63.8% of cases potentially relevant to interpretation because of missing data. This is a large percentage of cases to be losing because of missing data. It draws attention to the opportunities for improvement in the management of information.

Summary Observations

There comes a point in the interpretation of clinical performance data that collected raw data must be sorted and organized, or summarized, in a form that enables interpreters to begin to make sense of the data. Summarizing work involves developing frequency distributions and calculating for these distributions measures of central tendency and data spread. Measures of central tendency (for instance, the median) and dispersion (for instance, the interquartile range) allow comparison between two or more frequency distributions. When differences are observed between two distributions, interpreters are led to seek the reasons, or underlying factors, for the differences. Important points of this chapter are listed below.

1. Summarizing data is the process of expressing unsorted raw data in a form that will permit, directly or by means of further calculations, conclusions to be drawn.

2. A frequency distribution, or distribution, is the complete summary of the frequencies of the values or categories of measurement made on a group of entities.

3. A bell-shaped curve, or normal distribution, is an example of a distribution in which the greatest number of observations (measurements) falls in the center with fewer and fewer observations falling evenly on either side of the arithmetic average, or mean. Most data do not conform readily to a normal distribution. Rather, their distributions are skewed to the left or to the right.

4. The median, mean, and mode are three measures of central tendency for a distribution.

5. The median of a data set's distribution is the middle number when the measurements are arranged sequentially from smallest to largest or from largest to smallest. It is the most valid measure of central tendency whenever a distribution is skewed. It is often used in conjunction with the interquartile range.

6. The mean of a distribution specifies the arithmetic average—that is, the sum of all the measurements divided by the total number of measurements in the data set. The mean is best used as a measure of central tendency when the distribution of data is balanced, as in a normal curve, because the mean may be affected by large outlying measurements, such as in skewed, or asymmetric, distributions. The mean is often used in conjunction with the standard deviation.

7. Three measures of dispersion for a distribution are the range, the standard deviation, and the interquartile range.

8. The range is the distance between the lowest and highest values in a data set, calculated by subtracting the lowest value in the data set from the highest value in that same set. Its usefulness as a measure of dispersion is limited because it is based on only the two extreme values in a data set and ignores the distribution of all the values within those limits.

9. The standard deviation has a constant relationship with the area under a normal curve and is equal to the square root of the mean of all the squares of the deviations from the mean. It has two main purposes: to summarize the difference in distributions by measuring the variability of each distribution in a single number (statistic), and to enable data interpreters to test whether the differences in variability observed between two distributions are more than would be likely to have arisen by chance alone. The standard deviation's major limitation is that it is meaningless in non-normally distributed data. The standard deviation is often used in conjunction with the mean.

10. The interquartile range is a measure of dispersion around the median of a distribution and is most useful in describing non-normally distributed data. It involves dividing a distribution into four equal parts, or quartiles. A quartile's boundary is at the 25th, 50th, or 75th percentiles of such a distribution. The third quartile is the point below which 75% of the values lie. The interquartile range is the range in values between the first and third quartiles, designated Q1–Q3. The interquartile range is often used in conjunction with the median.

11. Sampling distributions are important in constructing and using control charts for attribute data.

References

1. Joint Commission on Accreditation of Healthcare Organizations: *Lexikon: Dictionary of Health Care Terms, Organizations, and Acronyms for the Era of Reform.* Oakbrook Terrace, IL: JCAHO, 1994, pp 263–264.

2. Hill AB: *Principles of Medical Statistics.* 9th ed. New York: Oxford University Press, 1971, p 60.

3. Joint Commission on Accreditation of Healthcare Organizations: *Lexikon: Dictionary of Health Care Terms, Organizations, and Acronyms for the Era of Reform.* Oakbrook Terrace, IL: JCAHO, 1994, p 455.

4. Ibid, p 453.

5. Ibid, p 484.

6. Ibid, p 750.

7. Rowntree D: *Statistics Without Tears: A Primer for Non-mathematicians.* New York: Charles Scribner's Sons, 1972, pp 72–78.

8. Burr IW: *Statistical Quality Control Methods.* New York: Marcel Dekker, 1976, p 32.

9. Rowntree D: *Statistics Without Tears: A Primer for Non-mathematicians.* New York: Charles Scribner's Sons, 1972, p 124.

10. Ibid, p 90.

CHAPTER SEVEN

Identifying Undesirable Data Variation

Recognizing and interpreting variation in clinical performance data is at the heart of data interpretation. It guides interpreters in making decisions concerning when to react, or not react, to specific data points or patterns of data. This chapter primarily focuses on Dr Walter Shewhart's theory and method for interpreting variation in processes, both within and across health care organizations.

Characterizing Variation

Variation is fluctuation in a series of results over time. When faced with variation, people tend to think about it in predictable ways. The most common way of thinking about variation is to assign a value judgment to its presence—that is, variation is either good or bad. For instance, variation in a hospital's indicator rate over time is commonly judged as either good (for example, moving toward some numerical goal) or bad (moving away from some numerical goal). Methods commonly used to determine whether variation is good or bad include "specifications, budgets, forecasts, numerical goals, and other tools for judging performance."[1]

This interpretation of variation can raise two important barriers to understanding. First, interpreting a series of results as good or bad does not provide information about the factors that underlie the observed variation. Second, this interpretation of variation tends to be suffused with emotion ("That is a bad rate! You are fired!" or "This is a great rate! You are promoted!").

A growing number of people are learning to think about variation in a new, more constructive way; variation observed in data falls into one of two categories: it is either common-cause variation or special-cause variation. An understanding of common causes and special causes of variation, as described below, provides a reasoned basis for action to improve a process of care or a patient health outcome.

Goal of Studying Variation in Clinical Performance Data

The immediate goal of studying variation in clinical performance data is to identify the occurrence of *unusual* variation. But what comprises unusual variation—that is, *what comprises variation to which interpreters should react?* Conversely, *what comprises variation for which interpreters can safely postpone or decide against any reaction?* These are the fundamental questions in all analyses of clinical performance data.

Is unusual variation in clinical performance data easily recognized? The answer is: not often. Indeed, variation of any kind or degree tends to create confusion. Amid the confusion, many people rely on common sense (their innate judgment) to determine whether observed variation is unusual. Unusual variation demands immediate action. Usual variation, by contrast, does not ordinarily require immediate action.

Common sense is not a reliable guide to determining whether variation is unusual because common sense commonly results in committing two fundamental types of errors. First, an interpreter may take action based on a reading that variation is unusual, when in reality the variation is usual and, therefore, no action is desirable.

This course of action wastes resources and can unnecessarily precipitate further variation, which then must be dealt with. Second, an interpreter may miss an opportunity for taking action (or learning what makes a process behave as it does) based on an interpretation that variation is usual, when in reality the variation is unusual and, therefore, action *should* be taken. This course of action can adversely affect patients' health.

Three Belief Systems About Variation

All people react to, and cope with, variation in their environment in distinctive ways. Bounds et al suggest that people use one of three major approaches to interpret the variation they encounter.[2]

Overreacting to Variation

One group of people believes that *all observed variation is the result of something exceptional, usually one obvious cause.* This cause, once identified, is analyzed in excruciating detail and acted on with vigor. This group of people does not understand that variation is inherent in the output of every dynamic system and that every observed fluctuation in output does not necessarily warrant reaction or action.

Taking action on some signal of variation without taking into account the difference between special-cause and common-cause variation is called *tampering*. Dr W. Edwards Deming illustrated tampering with his famous Funnel Experiment, which demonstrates by theory the losses that are caused by overreacting to variation.[3] Deming also opined that every suit for malpractice in medicine today operates on the thesis that somebody was at fault; that is, the event was due to some exceptional, or special, cause.[4]

Peter Senge also describes this kind of behavior. He calls it a "fixation on events," which is one of seven learning disabilities that may afflict organizations.[5] Managers, for example, who share this belief system look for a single, obvious explanation for an event each time it occurs and then make changes in the system to try to correct the cause they believe led to the event's occurrence. The managers fail to consider whether the event was due to the process itself or to a special cause. They may make the error of reacting to an outcome as if it came from some special cause, when actually it came from the system itself. The net result of this approach is increased, rather than decreased, variation.

Ignoring Variation

A second group of people believes that *variation should not exist as long as standards and practices, developed to produce uniform results, are scrupulously followed.* When any variation is observed, this group believes that the variation is the result of failing to comply with relevant standards and practices. The variation, this group argues, will disappear when compliance with standards is achieved. This group of people believes that worrying about variation is a waste of time and prefers instead to simply ignore it. When the desired level of performance is not achieved, the recourse is to deal more stringently with standards noncompliance.

There are at least three problems with this approach. *First, standards may be arbitrary or developed with insufficient information and knowledge of a system's capability to achieve prescribed results.* Deming's famous Red Bead Experiment illustrates this issue well.[6] In this experiment, "Willing Workers" can never meet the arbitrary goals (process specifications) set by the organization because the system in which they are asked to work is incapable of producing the output the organization unrealistically expects. Bounds et al state that "managing to arbitrary targets, rewarding or praising those who exceed them and penalizing or berating those who fail to meet them, is founded in the theory that variation should not exist."[2]

Second, forcing people to work toward meeting unrealistic standards can hurt outcomes. People may concentrate on complying with known standards—that is, those for which people believe they will be graded. Other important dimensions of performance that are not being monitored may be neglected. Workers may be fully aware that their efforts to improve a monitored dimension of performance is occurring at the expense of unmonitored dimensions. This approach to dealing with standards may eventually culminate in poor outcomes despite perfect compliance with monitored standards. This approach to coping with variation does not reliably improve, and may actually hurt, outcomes.

Third, ignoring variation can lead to lowering of workers' self-esteem. A worker who cannot meet expectations for process specifications, however unrealistic they may be, will not feel good about himself or herself. When workers become fearful and demoralized, the success of the organization becomes imperiled.

Walter Shewhart's Approach to Variation

A growing number of people are beginning to understand that *variation in results exists as a consequence of actions and interactions of the causes that produced the results.*[2] In the 1920s a young physicist named Dr Walter A. Shewhart working at Bell Telephone Laboratories invented this new way to think about uniformity and nonuniformity. His approach to variation centered on three discoveries.

First, he identified two sources of variation: variation arising from common causes and variation arising from special causes. As pointed out by Deming, "This in itself was a great contribution to knowledge."[7] Shewhart called them chance causes and assignable causes, now known as common causes and special causes, respectively.[7, 8] Deming popularized the terms "common cause" and "special cause."[9] Shewhart's original language is still used intermittently in the literature (for example, see Burr in *Statistical Quality Control Methods*).[8]

Second, Shewhart identified two kinds of mistakes, previously mentioned, made by people in the process of reacting to variation. The first mistake is to react to an outcome as if it came from a special cause, when actually it came from common causes of variation. The second mistake is to treat an outcome as if it came from common causes of variation, when actually it came from a special cause.

Third, Shewhart discovered and developed the control chart for interpreting variations in samples.

> Wrestling with a problem made complicated by presence of random variation, [Shewhart] came to realize that the problem was statistical in nature. Some of the observed variation in performance was natural to the process and unavoidable. But from time to time there would be variations which could not be so explained.

> [Shewhart] reached the brilliant conclusion that it would be desirable *and* possible to set limits upon the natural variation of any process, so that fluctuations within these limits would be readily explained by chance causes, but any variation outside this band would indicate a change in the underlying process.[10]

Shewhart laid out the whole field of statistical quality control, including its theory, philosophy, applications, and economic aspects, in his now famous *Economic Control of Quality of Manufactured Product*, which was published in 1931.[11] Burr notes that "few fields of knowledge have ever been so completely explored and charted in the first exposition."[10] The industrial field of quality control got its name from this book. A second book by Shewhart, *Statistical Method from the Viewpoint of Quality Control*, was published in 1939 with a foreword by Deming.[12]

Common-Cause Variation

Common-cause variation is fluctuation in a series of results that is due to the process and is produced by interactions of variables of that process. It is inherent in all processes.

Common causes of variation are the ever-present influences, or factors, that lie behind a particular measurement or result undergoing interpretation. Consider, for example, the seemingly simple process of documenting a seriously injured patient's arrival time at the emergency department. (Many of the Joint Commission's trauma care indicators rely heavily on this single data element.) Even when organizational staff try to hold all conditions as constant as possible, there are bound to be slight differences in the time or times recorded in the patient record.

For instance, the admitting clerk's watch may be slightly fast while the nurse's watch may be slightly slow. The clocks in the emergency department may be slow, fast, asynchronous, or temporarily broken, or they may be located so far away from patient care areas that reading them accurately (or at all) is challenging. The lighting in the emergency department may be inadequate in certain areas because it was designed that way or because burnt-out lightbulbs have not been replaced, making accurate reading of a watch or clock difficult. People may misread their watches for a variety of reasons even when the lighting is fine.

There may be several places in the patient record for recording arrival time depending on the function of the staff person making the entry—one place in the record designated for the admitting clerk, one for the nurse, and one more for the physician. The chart abstractor must decide which time (if, for instance, three different times are recorded) reflects the true time the patient arrived. The abstractor may not be able to locate the patient's arrival time even if it is present, buried deeply in a thick chart. Handwriting may not be legible. Some staff members may use military time, others not. Certain parts of the patient record containing arrival time may be missing.

All these influences and many others may each have a relatively minor effect, but taken together contribute to increased variability in the resulting measurements. This variability occurs even when an organization tries to hold all conditions as constant as is humanly possible. These influences add up to the natural variation inherent to every process. These influences are what is meant by common causes.

It is important to realize that common causes of variation are endogenous to a system and are not disturbances (they *are* the system) and that they can be removed or eliminated only by making basic changes in the system. For instance, if inadequate lighting, broken clocks, or messy charting is contributing to the documentation of inaccurate patient arrival times to the emergency department, the only way to eliminate these causes is to change the system for lighting the emergency department, change the system for providing the time of day for emergency department staff, and change the system for generating charts.

Deming offered a utilitarian definition of common-cause variation as the kind of variation that produces "points on a control chart that over a long period all fall inside the control limits. Common causes of variation stay the same day to day, lot to lot."[7]

There is no dearth of synonyms for the term *common cause*. As previously mentioned, Shewhart's original term was *chance cause*. Other synonyms include random cause, endogenous cause, and systemic cause.[8, 13]

Special-Cause Variation

Special-cause variation is the fluctuation in a series of results that is due to factors that intermittently and unpredictably induce variation over and above that inherent in a particular system.[14] Special causes of variation are *not* part of the process or system all the time or do not affect everyone, but arise because of specific circumstances.[15]

According to an article published in the *Wall Street Journal*,[16] a hospital that routinely monitored its intrahospital mortality rates for Medicare beneficiaries receiving coronary artery bypass graft (CABG) procedures noted some unusual and disturbing variation in its CABG mortality data. The 30-day hospital mortality rate for the bypass procedure had been below average (3%) for years, but began to worsen and finally increased to 7.6% at about the same time one of the hospital's two cardiovascular surgeons was confronted by hospital disciplinary bodies about substance abuse.

The second surgeon (recruited by the first) was confronted at the same time about his competence to perform bypass surgery based on new information about his past training. Later, when a new cardiovascular surgeon had replaced the former two, the mortality rate for bypass surgery fell to 1.5%, which was much better than the state average.

Although there was much discussion in this case about common causes, such as patient mix, that might be affecting the hospital's elevated CABG mortality rates, many people familiar with the case concluded that there was little doubt that substance abuse and incompetence were probably contributing to the increase in hospital CABG mortality rates. In this case, substance abuse and incompetence are two examples of special causes that probably affected the variation observed in the clinical performance data.

Deming defined special causes of variation as something special, not part of the system of common causes. They are detected any time a point falls outside the control limits of a control chart.[17]

Comparing Common and Special Causes of Variation

It is important to note that common and special causes are not always as easily distinguished as one might be led to believe. In reality, common and special causes are "more or less distinct" but "no hard and fast distinction can be made between them."[8] Probability can guide interpreters, however, as will be demonstrated in the following section on control charts.

There are several typical differences that can guide interpreters in making judgments as to whether a cause is common or special. Usually common causes are large in number, the effect of each is slight, and, on an individual basis, they may not be worth seeking out. Usually special causes are few in number (perhaps only one), the effect of each is marked, and they are well worth seeking out. In fact, they must be investigated without delay. To remove common causes means to fundamentally change the process. The most appropriate party to lead these changes is the manager(s) of the system. To remove special causes means to fix the process. The most appropriate party to perform this task is the workers who are intimately involved with the process.[8, 9]

Introduction to Shewhart Control Charts

A control chart is a graphic display of data in the order that they occur with statistically determined upper and lower limits of expected common-cause variation.[18] Shewhart devised the control chart to provide a consistent method to study variation within processes over time and to link variation to its sources, that is, common causes versus special causes. The control chart and its rules for use give interpreters an excellent means to make clear and repeatable judgments of statistical control of variation in the results. The primary advantage of using a control chart is to minimize the economic loss that comes from mistakes that occur in interpreting the meaning of variation.

To understand the advance in knowledge that Shewhart's discovery of control charts represents, it is helpful to examine the precursor to control charts, namely, run charts. *A run chart is a display of performance data in which data points are plotted as they occur over time to detect trends or other patterns and variation occurring over time.*[19] Run charts are commonly used today in health care to sequentially graph the rate of indicator occurrences over time. Figure 17 (see page 137), for instance, shows four such graphs for clinical performance indicators. Most readers would agree that all four graphs show variation. Beyond this observation, however, is a number of important questions:

- Which run chart seems to show the least variation or, alternatively, the greatest stability?
- Which run chart seems to show the greatest variation or, alternatively, the least stability?
- Which run chart seems to show variation stemming from random (chance) influences (that is, common causes)?

FIGURE 17 Run Charts for Four Performance Indicators

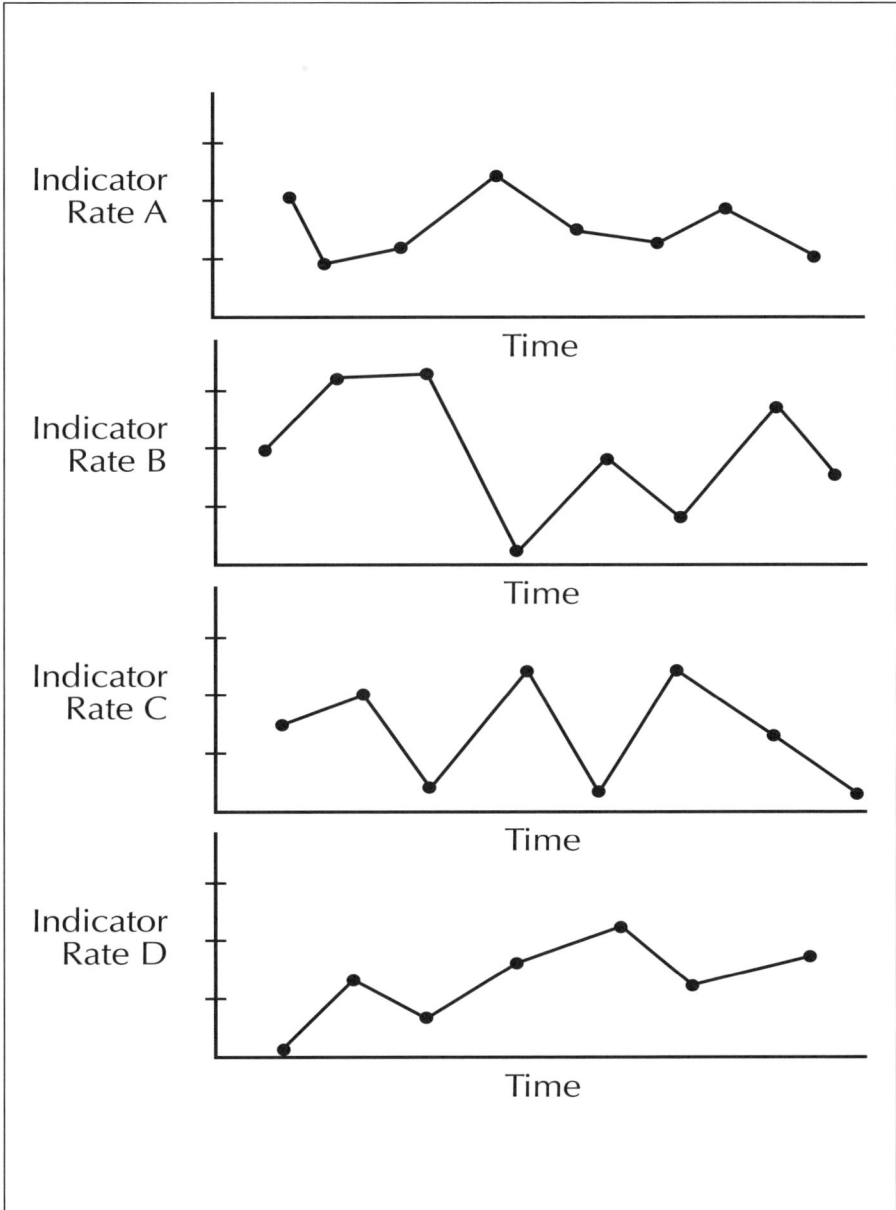

These four run charts show different patterns of variation. However, determining whether the variation comes from special causes or common causes is impossible, given just the information presented on these graphs.

- Which run chart seems to show variation stemming from special influences?
- Which of the graphs require us to act? Which of the graphs do not?

These are important questions to most interpreters because variation stemming from random influences (common causes) ordinarily requires no immediate action, whereas variation stemming from special causes does. *Yet, it is impossible to answer these questions from the information provided on the run charts.* Most health professionals who have had experience in interpreting run charts will agree that one of the most frustrating problems in studying run charts is trying to figure out what a high or low data point on a graph means. Shewhart's approach guides the interpreter to ask whether a high or low point on the graph indicates the presence of a special cause (which requires action), or whether a high or low point on the graph can so readily occur by common causes alone that there is no reliable evidence a special cause is present (and, therefore, no immediate action required). The way to ascertain the meaning of data points on a run chart is to rely on probability as a guide.

The basis of all control charts is that any varying quantity forms a frequency distribution if common causes alone are at work.[20] Any such distribution will also have a mean and a standard deviation. Burr explains that "quite regardless of the shape of the distribution (unless extremely badly behaved), there will be, by chance causes only, very few points outside of the band between the mean minus three standard deviations and the mean plus three standard deviations. Hence, having set such limits, we have a band of normal variability for the statistical measure in question." If a data point for one month lies outside the band of normal variability, Burr states:

> It is conceivable that such a point is just due to a rare "ganging up" of chance causes, and that no assignable cause was at work. But…it is a much better bet that the point outside the band is due to some assignable

cause. Hence when such a point comes along, we assume there was some assignable cause at work and try to see what process conditions might have changed.... Conversely, when a point lies inside the control band, we do not say that no assignable cause was present...but only that we have no reliable evidence for supposing that there was an assignable cause at work. Hence no action is taken. We attribute such points within the band as being due to chance causes only.

Thus, with control charts we save time looking for assignable causes when none are present and use this saved time for more careful search in those cases in which we do have reliable evidence of some nonchance factor at work.... The control chart is a most powerful tool for making more fruitful our efforts in stabilizing and controlling our processes at desired performances.[20]

Figure 18 (see page 140) shows the same run charts as shown in Figure 17, but now center lines and control limits have been added. The control limits are the boundaries for the upper and lower bands of normal variability. Now interpreters can readily ascertain which indicator rates are in control (Figures 18A and 18C) and which show evidence of special causes (Figures 18B and 18D).

Advantages of a Process in Good Control

There are five advantages to having a process brought into control.[20]

1. First, a process that is in control can be assumed to be free from sources of variation that are worth identifying. The process of care as currently designed and executed is doing all that can be expected of it. To improve on the process's output requires fundamental change in the process itself (that is, removing common causes).

For instance, the overall discrepancy rate between non-radiologists' interpretations of emergency department patients' x-rays

FIGURE 18 Control Charts for Four Performance Indicators Depicted in Figure 17

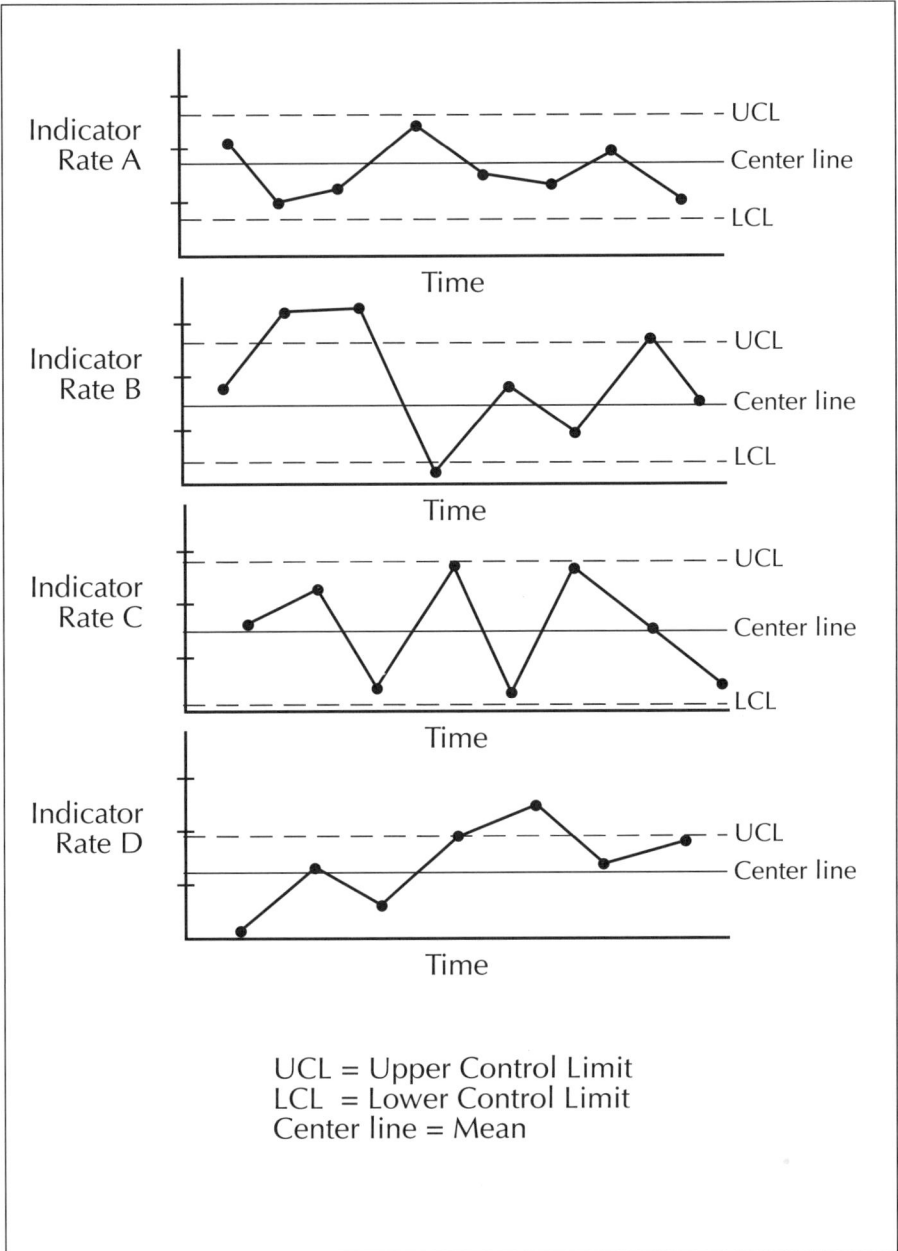

UCL = Upper Control Limit
LCL = Lower Control Limit
Center line = Mean

Adding center lines and control limits to the run charts in Figure 17 makes it possible to determine which patterns of indicator rates are in control and which suggest special causes.

is noted to be in control over time. Nonradiologists, such as emergency physicians, family practitioners, pediatricians, nurse practitioners, or physician assistants, may be required to perform x-ray interpretations for their patients when radiologists are not on site to interpret x-rays. The discrepancy rates range between 5% and 11% and no data points fall outside the band of normal variability on the control chart. This means that the observed data points can be reliably attributed to chance influences, or common causes, alone. The process for interpreting x-rays as designed and executed is doing about all that can be expected of it. If this range of discrepancy rates is unacceptable to the organization, the only way to improve the range is to make fundamental changes to the system, such as providing patients with 24-hour on-site coverage by radiologists or acquiring the means to transmit x-ray images from a site of care (such as an emergency department) to off-site radiologists for immediate interpretation and communication of results to providers at the site of care.

2. Second, getting a process into good statistical control ordinarily involves identifying and removing undesirable special causes and possibly including some good ones, such as new methods. For instance, a hospital is just beginning to monitor its performance taking vital signs of seriously injured trauma patients in the emergency department. For years, some staff members have been concerned with the emergency unit's performance of this process of care and have noted that the current structure of charts discourages staff from taking and documenting vital signs in an appropriate and timely manner. Staff have developed an improved chart with special areas designated for documenting frequent vital signs, including neurological measurements, to be used for the most seriously ill or injured patients cared for in the emergency department. The chart, however, has never been implemented because of complaints about its cost, inertia in getting the chart approved by appropriate hospital committees, and a multitude of other hitches.

After a brief period of monitoring how well vital signs are currently being taken, it becomes obvious to emergency department staff and hospital administrators that the process is, in a statistical sense, out of control. The new chart is approved and implemented, and subsequent measurements show that the process is in good control with no points falling outside the band of normal variability on the control chart. The special cause (poor charting instrument) has been removed and a good special cause (an improved charting instrument) has been added.

3. Third, any process that is in good control is predictable and stable. Variation is consistent, and the results fluctuate randomly around a steady average. Customers of the process know what to expect. If a health care plan, for instance, is monitoring the use of cancer staging by managing physicians and the process is in control, the rate will fluctuate randomly around some steady average (hopefully a relatively high average).

An out-of-control process, by contrast, will be unpredictable and unstable. Variation in an out-of-control process is inconsistent over time, shows a changing average, or shows no systematic pattern over time. Customers of the process never know what to expect. For instance, a patient does not know whether he or she will survive an operation if the surgical process is out of control in a statistical sense. Each time output is received, customers must inspect the output because they never know whether what they have received will be what they ordered. When a process is out of control (in a statistical sense), the organization must identify special causes and *eliminate them.*

It is important to reiterate that a process may be in good control in a statistical sense (that is, stable and predictable) but still not meet an organization's expectations or goals, either for the amount of variation or the mean performance. In this situation, many small common causes are resulting in unacceptable performance. The way to improve performance in this situation is through fundamental changes to the system.

4. Fourth, when a process is in good control, the output is

predictably known so that an organization can begin to offer assurances about the safety of the process. For instance, a hospital whose process for CABG surgery is in good control (the intrahospital mortality rate shows no data points outside the band of normal variability on the control chart over time) can provide important specific information to prospective patients about the relative safety of the procedure or, conversely, the risk of dying associated with the procedure.

5. Fifth, the best way to decrease the need for inspection is by bringing a process in control. Inspection involves measuring, examining, testing, or gauging one or more characteristics of an outcome and comparing these results with specified requirements to determine conformity. Inspection is a past-oriented strategy that attempts to identify unacceptable output after it has been produced and separate it from the good output.[21]

Inspection is also very expensive. Deming admonished people to cease dependence on mass inspection.[22] He asserted that "inspection with the aim of finding the bad ones and throwing them out is too late, ineffective, costly.... In the first place, you can't find the bad ones, not all of them. Second, it costs too much.... Quality comes not from inspection but from improvement of the process."[23]

Structure of a Control Chart

The structure of all control charts is similar. As depicted in Figure 18, each control chart has a center line representing the average of the process or outcome and an upper and a lower control limit that provide information on variation in the process or outcome over time.

Control charts are constructed by drawing samples, or subgroups, from some process or outcome undergoing measurement.[24] If a hospital is monitoring some process of care, clinical performance data related to this process are collected monthly. Each data point (indicator rate) relates to one subgroup. For Joint Commission beta indicators, each subgroup is composed of varying numbers of denominator cases for that indicator (see the section in this chapter on constructing a p chart).

Control limits are based on the variation that occurs within each subgroup. Variation between the subgroups is thus intentionally excluded from the calculation of the control limits.

Control limits must always be calculated with the assumption that no special causes of variation are influencing the system. Thus, the special causes (to the extent that they exist) have already been eliminated from the process, rendering the process in good control, as described in the previous section. Then, if a special cause begins to influence variation, the control chart, which is based solely on common variation, will show a data point that lies beyond the band of normal variability.

Control Chart Center Line

As described in Chapter Six, the center line of a control chart is equivalent to the mean of the sample means. For process or outcome indicators, the center line is equivalent to the mean proportion, which represents the average indicator rate for the reporting period shown on the chart. Calculation of the center line value is described in the section on constructing a *p* chart.

Upper and Lower Control Limits

The upper control limit is equal to the mean plus three times the estimated standard error. The lower control limit is equal to the mean minus three times the estimated standard error. Recall from Chapter Six that the standard error is a measure of the deviation of a sampling distribution. It enables interpreters to calculate the chances that a particular sample mean will be much larger or smaller than the process (or outcome) average. Calculation of control limits is described in the section on constructing a *p* chart.

Categories of Control Charts

Control charts can be divided into two broad categories: variables control charts and attribute control charts. *Variables control charts* are composed of *variables data*, which are measurements such as weight, length, width, time, and temperature. *Attribute control charts* are composed of *attribute data*, which arise from classifying items into categories, for instance, indicator occurrence or nonoccurrence (see Chapters Four and Six). The cardiovascular, oncology, and trauma care indicators tested by the Joint Commission with beta-testing hospitals produced attribute data, which are the focus of the following discussion.

Attribute Control Charts (*p* Charts)

Although there are three types of attribute control charts, we are concerned here only with the *binomial count chart*, commonly known as the *p* chart.[24] The *p* chart deals with the fraction of items in a series of subgroups that have a certain characteristic. For instance, an indicator rate of 50% for a subgroup measured for the month of May is an example of such a fraction. Subgroup sizes in a *p* chart may remain constant or may vary, as with the Joint Commission's beta indicators.

Constructing a *p* Chart

Several steps are involved in constructing a *p* chart for individual beta indicators.[25] *First, the manner, size, and frequency of subgroup selection must be established.* The size of subgroups for a given Joint Commission beta indicator, for example, varied depending on how many denominator (Category IV, see Chapter Six) cases a hospital transmitted during a given time period.

Second, the indicator rate must be calculated for each subgroup of denominator cases and then graphed. If a process of care is being monitored monthly, the mean indicator rate for data collected for each month must be calculated and plotted. As described in Chapter Six, if 50 denominator (Category IV) cases and 25 numerator (Category V) cases were collected for one month, the indicator rate for that month would be:

$$\frac{V}{IV + V} = \frac{25}{50 + 25} = .33 \ (33\%)$$

Table 12 (see page 147) lists monthly indicator rates for a hospital monitoring some process of care or patient health outcome. Figure 19 (see page 148) shows these data points graphed on a chart.

Third, the center line, which is the overall average indicator rate for a given reporting period, must be calculated from the data using the following equation:

$$\text{Center line } (\bar{p}) = \bar{p} = \frac{\text{Number of indicator occurrences}}{\substack{\text{Number in the population} \\ \text{described by the indicator}}}$$

If the total number of cases among subgroups in the population described by the indicator were 100 during a given reporting period (that is, Category IV plus Category V cases) and 41 cases of those 100 met the criteria for defining an indicator occurrence (that is, Category V cases), the mean proportion (center line) would calculate to .41 (41%). This center line value has been added to the chart in Figure 20 (see page 149). Because the mean proportion is the average for all months, its value does not vary from month to month as does the size of the denominator for each subgroup.

Fourth, control limits must be calculated and then plotted on the chart. The upper control limit is equal to the mean plus three times the estimated standard error. The lower control limit is equal to the mean minus three times the estimated standard error. The formula for calculating the standard error for a particular month is:

$$\text{Standard error for month } = \sqrt{\frac{\bar{p}(1-\bar{p})}{n}}$$

where p is the overall indicator rate and n is the denominator population for the month. The formula for the upper control limit (UCL) is:

UCL = p + 3(standard error for a given month).

The formula for the lower control limit (LCL) is:

LCL = p − 3(standard error for a given month).

Because the size of the denominator population varies from month

TABLE 12 Sample Rates for Cardiovascular Indicator 9

Monitoring Period	Hospital's Indicator Occurrence Rate
January	30%
February	42%
March	38%
April	39%
May	51%
June	16%

to month, the measure of variation (that is, the UCL and LCL) will also vary from month to month. Figure 21 (see page 150) depicts the chart with upper and lower control limits added to it (hatched lines). Note that these control limits vary from month to month. With the center line and control limits added, the chart has become a control chart.

Using a Control Chart to Study Variation

Once a control chart has been constructed, it is then examined for indications of a lack of control—that is, that the process or outcome is unstable. Recall that data points lying outside the normal band of variability (beyond the control limits) indicate that the process or outcome is out of control, that special causes of variation are likely in play, and that action is required to identify and eliminate the special causes.

The exact probabilities that a stable process will generate points indicating a lack of control are generally difficult to calculate for a p chart.[26] Gitlow et al point out that the exact value of these probabilities is not as important as the fact that they are very small. Thus, if a point does lie beyond the band of normal variability, it can be inferred that the process lacks control.

p charts have another useful dimension. Interpreters are not

FIGURE 19 Chart for Cardiovascular Indicator 9 with Monthly Indicator Rates and Subgroup Sizes Charted

---

Joint Commission: Beta Reports for Cardiovascular Indicators

Reporting Period: January 1, 1992 – June 30, 1992

Indicator
Occurrence
Rate

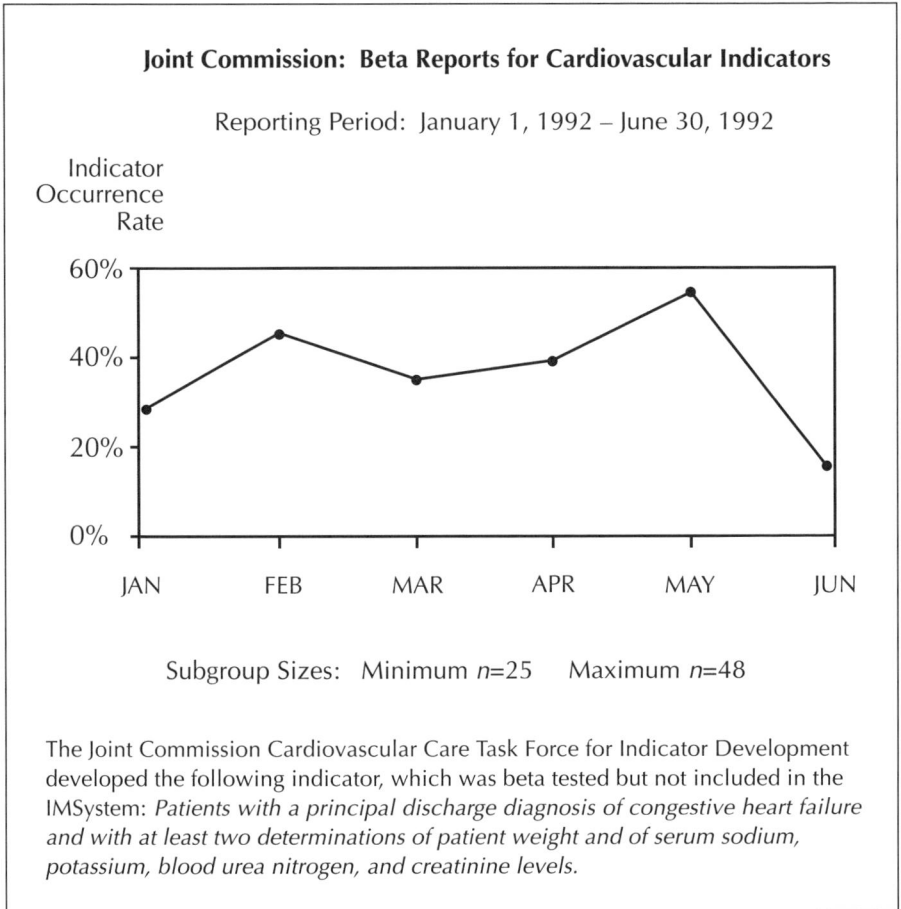

Subgroup Sizes: Minimum *n*=25   Maximum *n*=48

The Joint Commission Cardiovascular Care Task Force for Indicator Development
developed the following indicator, which was beta tested but not included in the
IMSystem: *Patients with a principal discharge diagnosis of congestive heart failure
and with at least two determinations of patient weight and of serum sodium,
potassium, blood urea nitrogen, and creatinine levels.*

This run chart graphs the indicator rates listed in Table 12, the second step
in constructing a *p* chart.

limited to searching for data points that lie beyond the control limits
to identify the existence of special causes of variation. *A process can
lack statistical control even when all data points are within control
limits but exhibit certain patterns of variation.*[27, 28]

Stable processes always exhibit random patterns of variation—
that is, as many points will fall above the mean as below the mean
over time and most points will tend to cluster closely about the

FIGURE 20 Chart for Cardiovascular Indicator 9 with Center Line (Mean Proportion) Added

Joint Commission: Beta Reports for Cardiovascular Indicators

Reporting Period: January 1, 1992 – June 30, 1992

Indicator
Occurrence
Rate

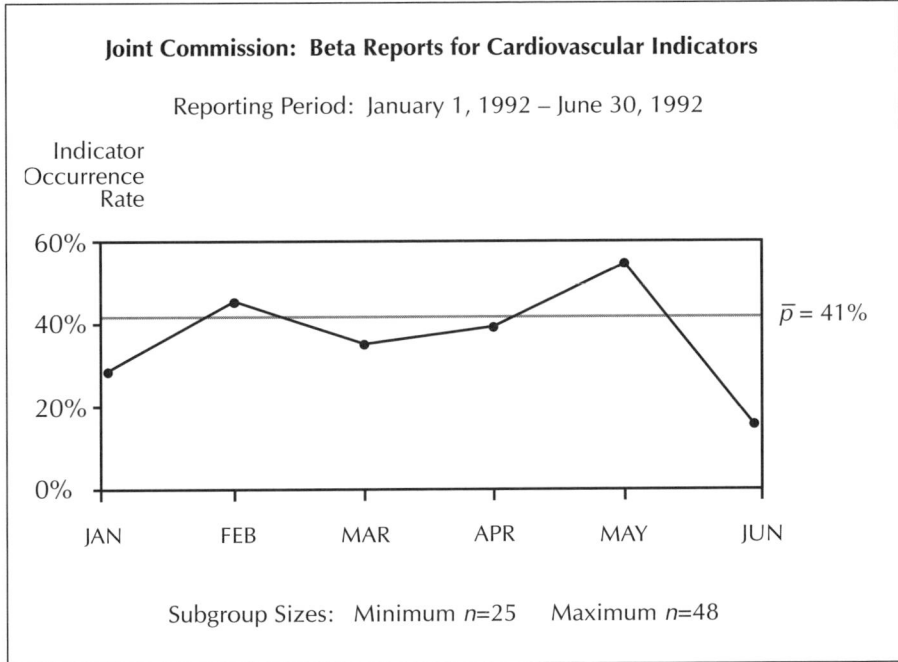

$\bar{p} = 41\%$

JAN   FEB   MAR   APR   MAY   JUN

Subgroup Sizes: Minimum *n*=25   Maximum *n*=48

The third step in constructing a *p* chart is calculating the center line, or average indicator rate for a given reporting period. In this example, the center line is 41 (41%) for the period January through June 1992.

center line. A departure from this random pattern of variation within the band of normal variability (that is, between control limits) suggests that nonrandom variation is occurring. For instance, a prolonged run of data points upward for eight consecutive subgroups would suggest that nonrandom variation is occurring because one would expect equal numbers of data points to fall above and below the mean over time and data points to be clustered about the mean if variation is truly random.

To identify patterns of data that signal a lack of control, the area between the upper and lower control limits on a control chart must be divided into six bands, or zones.[27] *Each zone is one standard error wide; C zones* correspond to one standard error on either side

FIGURE 21 Control Chart for Cardiovascular Indicator 9 with Control Limits Added

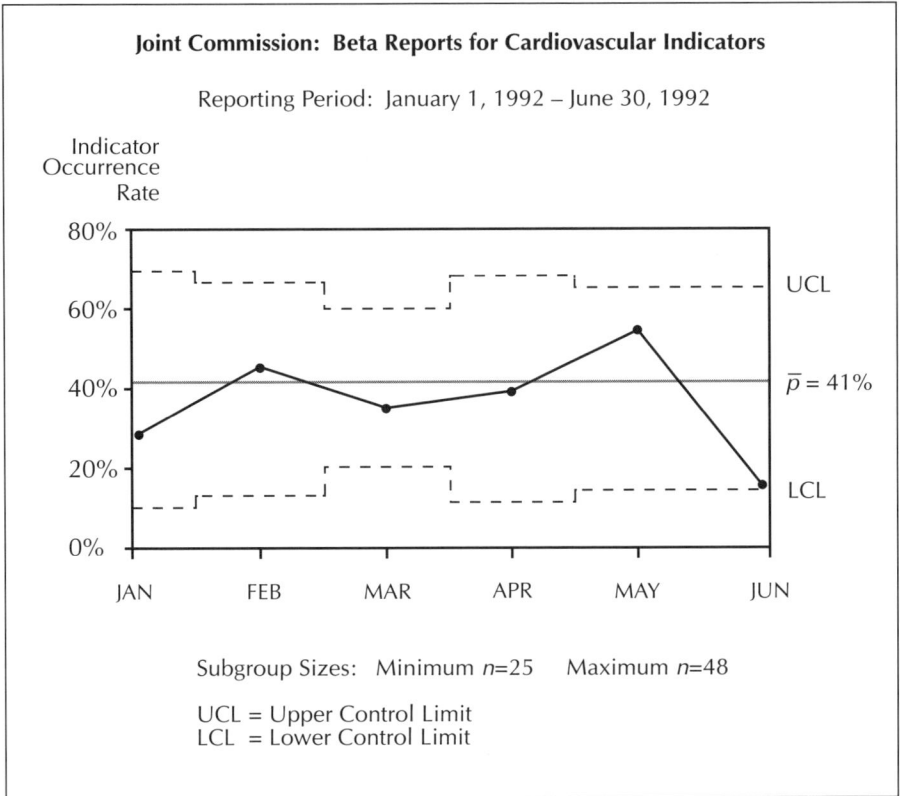

Joint Commission: Beta Reports for Cardiovascular Indicators

Reporting Period: January 1, 1992 – June 30, 1992

Indicator Occurrence Rate

UCL

$\bar{p} = 41\%$

LCL

JAN FEB MAR APR MAY JUN

Subgroup Sizes: Minimum n=25 Maximum n=48

UCL = Upper Control Limit
LCL = Lower Control Limit

The final step in constructing a *p* chart is calculating the upper control limit (UCL) and lower control limit (LCL). Note that the control limits vary from month to month.

of the center line, *B zones* correspond to two standard errors from the center line, and *A zones* correspond to the outermost bands (see Figure 22, page 151). Gitlow et al cite four rules based on A, B, and C zones that can help interpreters decide whether a process or outcome is exhibiting a lack of control despite all the data points falling within control limits:[27]

1. *A process or outcome demonstrates lack of control if any two of three consecutive points fall in one of the A zones or beyond on the same side of the center line.* Figure 23 (see page 152) depicts the first rule.

FIGURE 22 Six Control Chart Zones

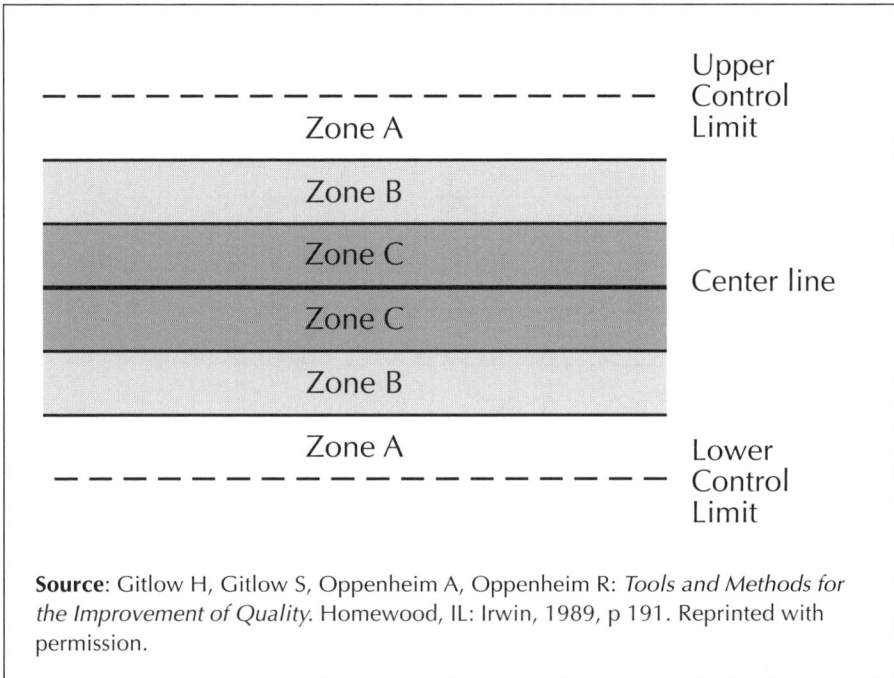

Zone A — Upper Control Limit

Zone B

Zone C — Center line

Zone C

Zone B

Zone A — Lower Control Limit

Source: Gitlow H, Gitlow S, Oppenheim A, Oppenheim R: *Tools and Methods for the Improvement of Quality*. Homewood, IL: Irwin, 1989, p 191. Reprinted with permission.

A control chart may be divided into six zones between the upper control limit (UCL) and the lower control limit (LCL). Each zone is one standard error wide.

2. *A process or outcome exhibits lack of control if four of five consecutive points fall in one of the B zones or beyond on the same side of the center line.* The second rule is shown in Figure 24 (see page 153).

3. *A process or outcome exhibits lack of control if eight or more consecutive points lie on one side of the center line.* Figure 25 (see page 154) demonstrates this third rule.

4. *A process or outcome demonstrates lack of control if eight or more consecutive points move upward or downward in value.* This fourth rule is shown in Figure 26 (see page 155).

5. *The Memory Jogger II* cites fifth and sixth rules:[28] *A process lacks control if 14 consecutive points alternate up and down* (see Figure 27, page 156). *A process lacks control if 15 consecutive points fall in zone C* (see Figure 28, page 157). *The Memory Jogger II* also

FIGURE 23 Out-of-Control Evidence on Control Charts: First Rule

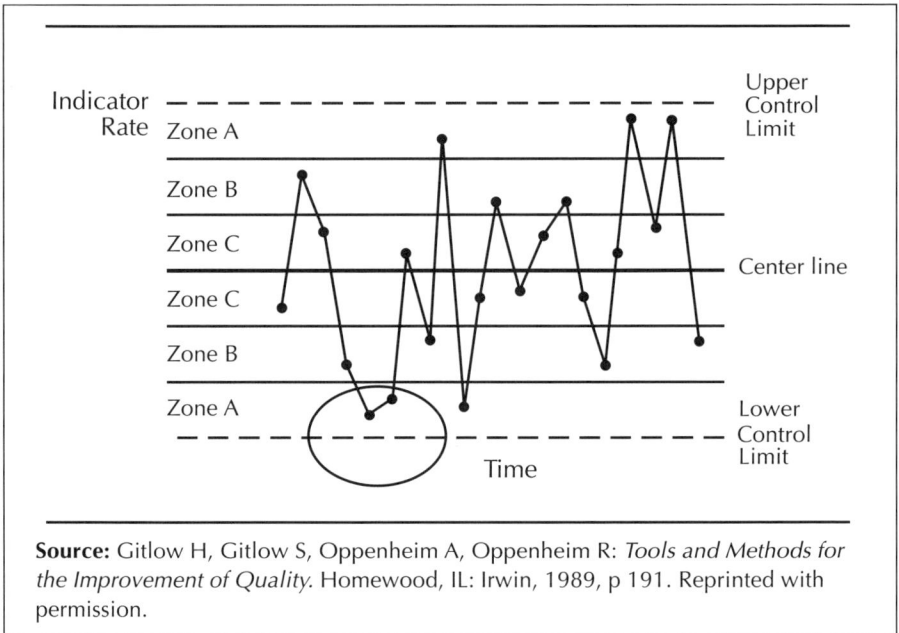

Source: Gitlow H, Gitlow S, Oppenheim A, Oppenheim R: *Tools and Methods for the Improvement of Quality.* Homewood, IL: Irwin, 1989, p 191. Reprinted with permission.

First rule: A process or outcome demonstrates lack of control if any two of three consecutive points fall in one of the A zones or beyond on the same side of the center line.

specifies the number seven, rather than eight, consecutive points for the third and fourth rules cited by Gitlow et al.

Variation Among Health Care Organizations and the Use of Comparison Charts

The focus of Chapter Seven thus far has been variation of a process or outcome within an organization over time. However, many interpreters express a keen interest in comparing an individual organization's clinical performance data with data calculated for other organizations. For instance, a hospital may have an indicator rate of 40% for a reporting period and want to know how this rate compares to the rates of peer hospitals using the identical indicator and indicator measurement system.

FIGURE 24 Out-of-Control Evidence on Control Charts: Second Rule

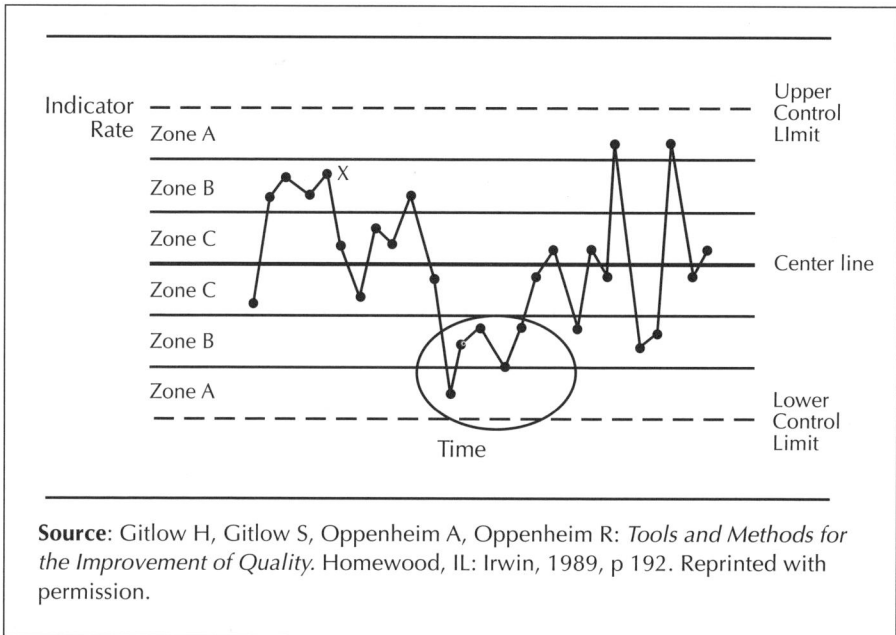

Source: Gitlow H, Gitlow S, Oppenheim A, Oppenheim R: *Tools and Methods for the Improvement of Quality.* Homewood, IL: Irwin, 1989, p 192. Reprinted with permission.

Second rule: A process or outcome exhibits lack of control if four of five consecutive points fall in one of the B zones or beyond on the same side of the center line.

There are two important issues concerning comparison of an organization's data to the data produced by one or more other organizations. First, the process or outcome must demonstrate good control across all organizations undergoing comparison before attempting to understand variation observed among organizations. If special causes of variation over time are influencing individual organization rates, comparisons among organizations should be made with caution or not at all.

Second, patient populations in different organizations may differ in a number of characteristics, such as average age. These patient characteristics may affect indicator rates. For instance, the mortality associated with a given procedure may increase with increased age.

Factors that differ between comparison groups and influence

FIGURE 25 Out-of-Control Evidence on Control Charts: Third Rule

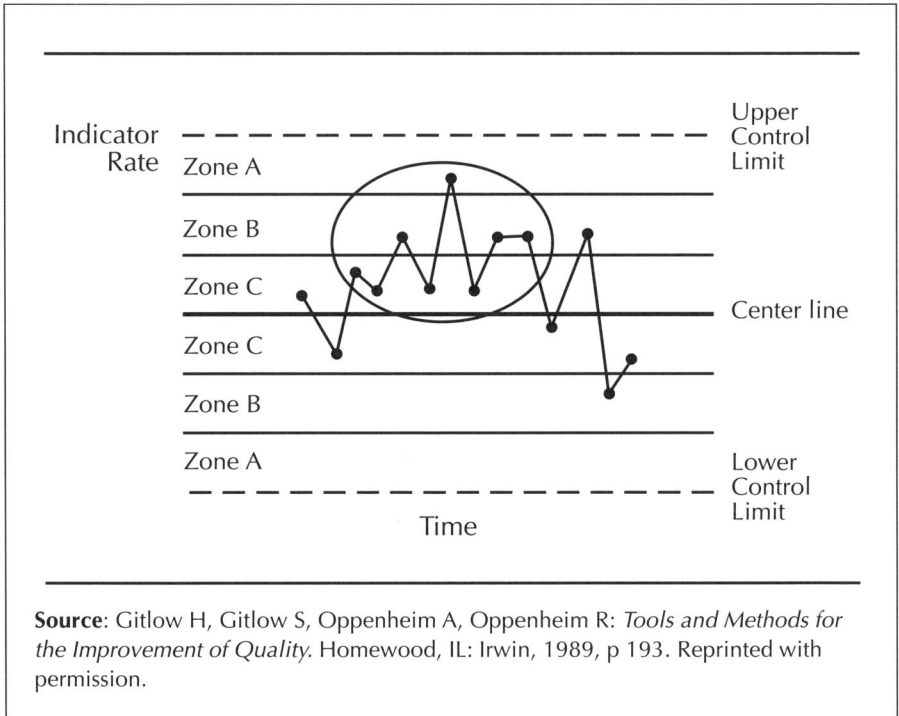

Source: Gitlow H, Gitlow S, Oppenheim A, Oppenheim R: *Tools and Methods for the Improvement of Quality.* Homewood, IL: Irwin, 1989, p 193. Reprinted with permission.

Third rule: A process or outcome exhibits lack of control if eight or more consecutive points lie on one side of the center line.

outcomes of interest are known as *confounding factors.* Unless the effects of confounding factors are statistically eliminated or reduced, comparisons will yield biased results. In other words, differences in patient populations among comparison hospitals, unless statistically dealt with, will lead to erroneous interpretation.

The statistical process used to overcome the effect of differences that can influence indicator rates, especially for outcomes, and distort comparison is called *risk adjustment.*

Risk Adjustment

Risk-adjustment techniques are statistical methods of analysis that attempt to control for bias due to confounding factors. Risk adjustment

FIGURE 26 Out-of-Control Evidence
on Control Charts: Fourth Rule

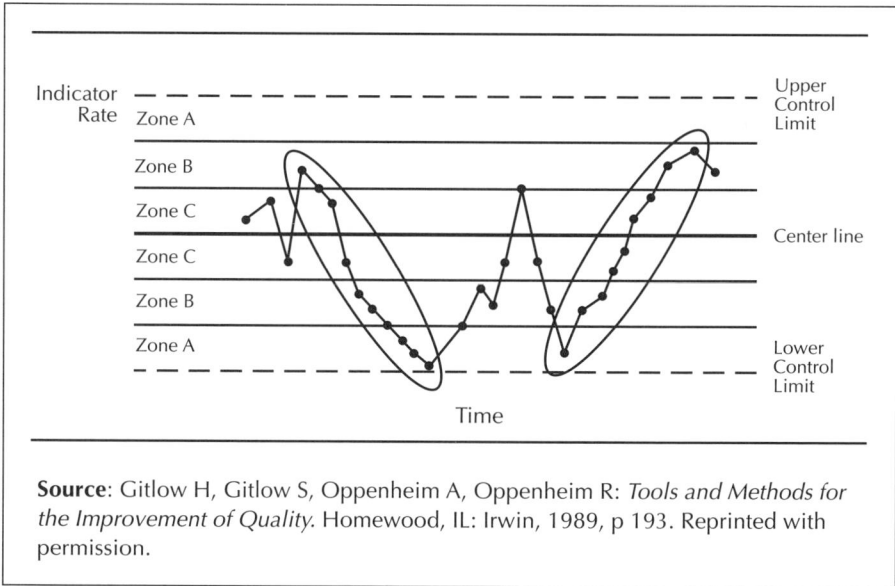

Source: Gitlow H, Gitlow S, Oppenheim A, Oppenheim R: *Tools and Methods for the Improvement of Quality.* Homewood, IL: Irwin, 1989, p 193. Reprinted with permission.

Fourth rule: A process or outcome demonstrates lack of control if eight or more consecutive points move upward or downward in value.

allows interpreters to estimate what would have happened if both comparison groups had been the same when, in fact, they were not. That is, the estimate of the difference between the two comparison groups is adjusted to compensate for the differences between the groups on the confounding factors.

In the Joint Commission's set of cardiovascular care beta indicators, the data are risk adjusted for various combinations of patient characteristics, such as age, gender, admission source, admission type, tobacco dependency, transfer from another hospital, type of angina, initial CABG, emergency CABG, and many others. The confounding factors for the Joint Commission's set of trauma care beta indicators include age, gender, injury severity score, and preexisting conditions, such as hypertension or alcohol/drug dependence.

The data produced by the beta-testing process are attribute data, which arise from classifying items into categories, as in indicator

FIGURE 27 Out-of-Control Evidence on Control Charts: Fifth Rule

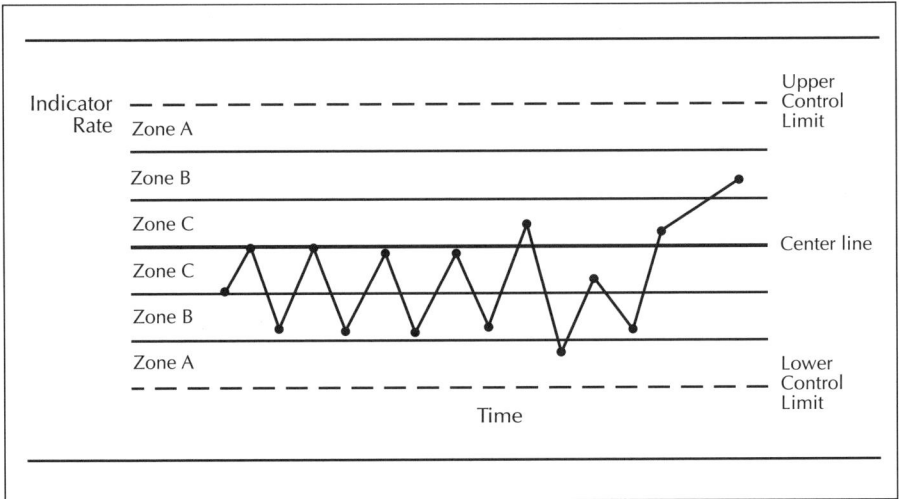

Fifth rule: A process or outcome lacks control if 14 consecutive points alternate up and down

occurrence or nonoccurrence. The confounding factors listed above are a mixture of attribute and variables data. Variables data come from measuring some characteristic, such as weight or time, on a continuous scale. To account for this situation, the statistical method used to risk adjust is *logistic regression*, or logit analysis.

Logistic Regression Model

A thorough understanding of the logistic regression model's methodology for risk adjustment and its application to comparison charts (described in the section on control charts) is not required in order to make productive use of comparison charts in comparing clinical performance data among organizations reporting to a common database. However, a brief description of logistic regression is presented here for interested readers.[29]

In the context of indicator measurement, *a logistic regression model is one way of describing the relationship between the probability of an outcome and a set of confounding variables* (for example,

FIGURE 28 Out-of-Control Evidence on Control Charts: Sixth Rule

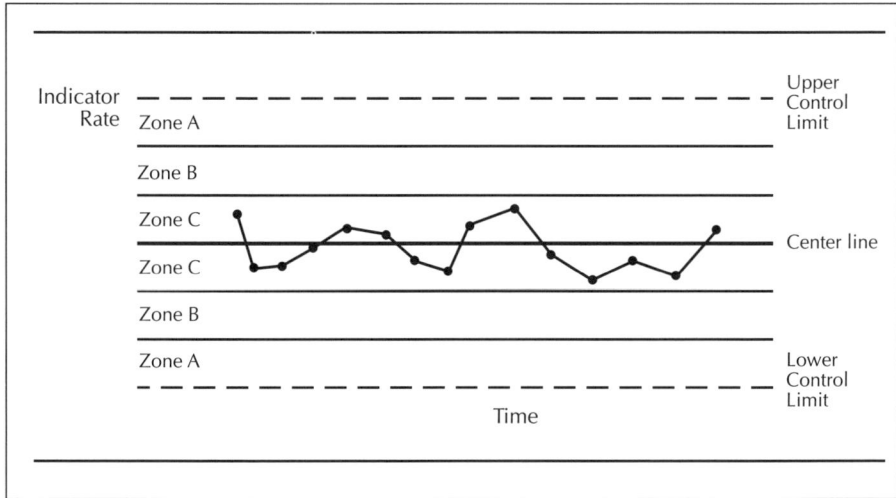

Sixth rule: A process or outcome lacks control if 15 consecutive points fall in zone C.

demographics, preexisting conditions, severity of injury). The usefulness of the logistic regression model is its ability to adjust for many confounding variables simultaneously. For any particular outcome indicator, only those confounding variables demonstrating a significant effect on the outcome are retained in the model. Therefore, each indicator studied will generate a separate logistic regression model.

Once the relationship between the outcome and confounding variables is estimated, the equation obtained can be used to calculate a predicted probability of outcome for an indicator patient, given a set of values for the confounding variables. To obtain a hospital's predicted indicator rate, these individual predicted probabilities are averaged over all the patients at risk for a particular indicator occurrence.

The calculation of the prediction range depends on the variation in the difference between the hospital's observed indicator rate and the indicator rate predicted from the logistic regression model. The variation in turn has at least three major components:

1. The first component of the variation, known as the model variance, results from the fitting of the logistic regression model. Since the logistic regression model is only an approximate description of the data available, variation is expected as a result of using the statistical model to fit the data.

2. The second component results from the variation in the observed indicator rate, known as the binomial variance. This type of variation results from estimating any indicator rate. For instance, this type of variation is used to calculate the control limits on a *p* chart.

3. The third component is the variation among hospitals not explained by the logistic regression model. This component basically captures the variation in the data not explained by the first two components.

The overall variation used in constructing the prediction range is the sum of these three components of variation.

Computation of the prediction range must account for the skewness that is inherent in any expected indicator rate that deviates far from 50%. Skewness may be thought of as a measure of how much the distribution of a variable deviates from the normal bell-shaped curve pattern. The prediction intervals used in a comparison chart are adjusted to account for skewness.

Structure of Comparison Charts

Comparison charts are visual devices used to compare the indicator rates among organizations reporting clinical performance data to a common performance database (Figure 29; see page 159). The data used for comparison charts must be risk adjusted to account for the differences between one hospital and the others on the confounding patient characteristics. If risk adjustment has not been performed for data, comparison charts should not be used.

The structure of all comparison charts is similar. As depicted in Figure 29, each comparison chart has two axes, a solid dot, cross hairs, and a vertical bar.

FIGURE 29 Example of a Comparison Chart

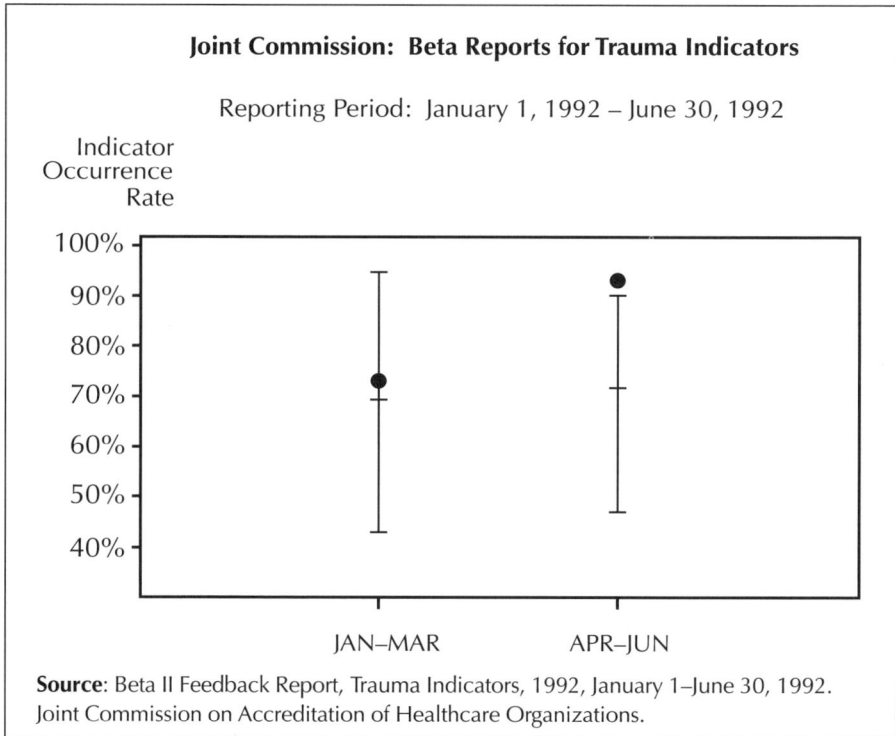

Joint Commission: Beta Reports for Trauma Indicators

Reporting Period: January 1, 1992 – June 30, 1992

Indicator
Occurrence
Rate

JAN–MAR   APR–JUN

Source: Beta II Feedback Report, Trauma Indicators, 1992, January 1–June 30, 1992.
Joint Commission on Accreditation of Healthcare Organizations.

This chart compares rates on the timeliness of patient transfers among
organizations reporting to the same database.

Axes

The *vertical axis* corresponds to indicator rate and the *horizontal
axis* corresponds to time. Indicator rates along the vertical axis
generally extend from 0 to 1 (0% to 100%). For some indicators,
however, the vertical axis may use only a portion of the entire scale
(for instance, from .02 to .10) depending on the range of indicator
rates unique to a particular indicator.

Solid Dot

The *solid dot* appearing above each quarterly block of months on
the horizontal scale represents the actual indicator rate observed for
a given beta-testing hospital. The dot shows the indicator rate

calculated from the data provided by the hospital for the reporting period indicated along the horizontal axis.

Cross Hairs

There are three horizontal *cross hairs* on the vertical bar. The *central cross hair* represents the indicator rate that would be predicted for a given hospital based on the cumulative experience of all patients in the total population (for example, the total beta hospital population). This predicted indicator rate is based on a statistical risk-adjustment model, as described earlier. The model takes into account patient characteristics influencing the indicator rate but not related to the quality of care provided by organizations. Cross hairs at the ends of the vertical bar simply represent the upper and lower points on the vertical bar itself. The cross hair may not be at the midpoint of the vertical bar because the distribution of rates in the overall population is not usually a normal distribution, but is skewed.

Vertical Bars

A vertical bar appears above each block of months. The length of the bar represents the 95% confidence interval of the predicted indicator rate. The confidence interval is based on the variation that would be expected to occur about the predicted value, based on the number of patients from a hospital used to calculate the observed indicator rate. The confidence interval is also based on the variation of the statistical adjustment model determined from the entire population.

If the observed rate shown by the solid dot is not on the vertical line, there is only a 5% probability that the difference between observed and predicted rates could be that extreme by chance alone. Such a small probability is unlikely and indicates that there is some systemic reason(s) why the observed rate fell outside the prediction interval. Systemic reasons for the difference may include organizational and/or practitioner performance issues.

Using a Comparison Chart to Study Variation

Comparison charts allow interpreters to directly compare one organization's indicator rate (shown by the solid dot) with that of all other organizations contributing to the database. The data have been risk adjusted to eliminate differences attributed solely to patient mix (that is, differences among patients receiving care at different institutions).

It is important to remember that comparison chart interpretations will be accurate only if the indicator rates shown on the comparison chart are stable over time. Stability can be determined from examination of the indicator's control chart.

Combined Use of Comparison Charts and Control Charts

Interpreters should be alerted when the monthly indicator rates of an organization are stable (that is, in good control), yet the overall quarterly rates fall outside the prediction interval on the indicator's comparison chart. This means that the particular process for a given organization is operating at a rate significantly different from other organizations contributing to the performance database.

This is extremely useful information. A given organization's process may be in perfect control over time, demonstrated by indicator data points on the control chart within the control limits and no suspicious out-of-control patterns. The organization does not take action on the data because there is no reliable evidence for supposing that special causes are at work. The data points within the control limits are due to chance causes only.

However, being in control does not necessarily mean that the process is meeting the needs of its customers. It only means that the process is consistent. Indeed, the process may be consistently mediocre or even consistently bad. The comparison chart can identify when an organization's rates are in control over time but bear little relationship to the rates reported by other organizations contributing to the database. This discrepancy directs attention to the possibility that an in-control process may require process improvement (fundamental changes). Improving in-control processes is discussed further in Chapter Eight.

Summary Observations

The study of variation in clinical performance data is the heart of the interpretation process. Important insights from this chapter are listed below.

1. Variation is fluctuation in a series of results over time. Variation is the inescapable product, or output, of any system or process. Variation in results, according to Dr Walter Shewhart, exists as a consequence of actions and interactions of the causes that produced the results.

2. Shewhart made three important discoveries about variation: (1) He identified two sources of variation—common causes and special causes; (2) he identified two kinds of mistakes made by people reacting to variation—reacting to an outcome as if it came from a special cause, when actually it came from common causes, and treating an outcome as if it came from common causes, when actually it came from a special cause; and (3) he discovered and developed the control chart for interpreting variations in samples, or subgroups.

3. Tampering is taking action on some signal of variation without taking into account the difference between special-cause and common-cause variation.

4. Common-cause variation is fluctuation in a series of results that is due to the process and is produced by interactions of variables of that process. It is inherent in all processes.

5. Special-cause variation is fluctuation in a series of results that is due to factors that intermittently and unpredictably induce variation over and above that inherent in a particular system. Special causes of variation are *not* part of the process or system all the time or do not affect everyone, but arise because of specific circumstances.

6. A control chart is a graphic display of data in the order that they occur with statistically determined upper and lower limits of expected common-cause variation. A control chart is used to indicate special causes of variation, to monitor a process for maintenance, and to determine if process changes have had the desired effect. The primary advantage of using a control chart is to minimize the economic loss that comes from mistakes that occur in interpreting the meaning of variation.

7. Variables control charts are composed of variables data, which are measurements such as weight, length, width, time, and temperature. Attribute control charts—also called *p* charts—are composed of attribute data, which arise from the classifying items into categories, for instance, indicator occurrence or nonoccurrence. The *p* chart deals with the fraction of items in a series of subgroups that have a certain characteristic.

8. Data points lying outside the normal band of variability (beyond the control limits) on a control chart indicate that the process or outcome is out of control, that special causes of variation are likely in play, and that action is required to identify and eliminate the special causes.

9. There are at least six out-of-control data patterns that can be observed *within* the band of normal variability.

10. Whenever data between organizations is being compared, two conditions must be met. First, the process or outcome must demonstrate good control before attempting to understand variation observed among organizations. Second, confounding factors that differ between comparison groups and influence outcomes of interest must be statistically eliminated or reduced, or comparisons will yield biased results. The statistical process used to overcome the effect of differences that can influence indicator rates and distort comparison is called risk adjustment.

11. Comparison charts are visual devices used to compare the indicator rates among organizations reporting clinical performance data to a common performance database.

References

1. Nolan TW, Provost LP: Understanding variation. *Quality Progress*, May 1990, pp 70–78.

2. Bounds G, Yorks L, Adams M, et al: *Beyond Total Quality Management: Toward the Emerging Paradigm.* New York: McGraw-Hill, 1994, pp 353–355.

3. Deming WE: *The New Economics for Industry, Government, Education.* Cambridge, MA: Massachusetts Institute of Technology Center for Advanced Engineering Study, 1993, pp 194–209.

4. Ibid, p 193.

5. Senge P: *The Fifth Discipline: The Art and Practice of the Learning Organization.* New York: Doubleday Currency, 1990, p 21.

6. Deming WE: *The New Economics for Industry, Government, Education.* Cambridge, MA: Massachusetts Institute of Technology Center for Advanced Engineering Study, 1993, pp 158–175.

7. Ibid, p 178.

8. Burr I: *Statistical Quality Control Methods.* New York: Marcel Dekker, 1976, pp 26–28.

9. Nolan TW, Provost LP: Understanding variation. *Quality Progress*, May 1990, pp 70–78.

10. Burr I: *Statistical Quality Control Methods.* New York: Marcel Dekker, 1976, p 29.

11. Shewhart WA: *Economic Control of Quality of Manufactured Product.* New York: Van Nostrand, 1931.

12. Shewart WA: *Statistical Method from the Viewpoint of Quality Control.* New York: Dover, 1986 (unabridged republication of the work originally published by the Graduate School of the Department of Agriculture, Washington, DC, 1939).

13. Joint Commission on Accreditation of Healthcare Organizations: *Lexikon: Dictionary of Health Care Terms, Organizations, and Acronyms for the Era of Reform,* Oakbrook Terrace, IL: JCAHO, 1994, p 198.

14. Ibid, pp 742–743.

15. Nolan TW, Provost LP: Understanding variation. *Quality Progress*, May 1990, pp 70–78.

16. Anders G: How 2 top surgeons saw lucrative practice collapse in acrimony: Million-dollar MDs lost it, one to alcohol and one, in part, to a past error. *Wall Street Journal* (southwest edition), Sep 13, 1994, pp A1, A8.

17. Deming WE: *The New Economics for Industry, Government, Education.* Cambridge, MA: Massachusetts Institute of Technology Center for Advanced Engineering Study, 1993, p 179.

18. Joint Commission on Accreditation of Healthcare Organizations: *Lexikon: Dictionary of Health Care Terms, Organizations, and Acronyms for the Era of Reform,* Oakbrook Terrace, IL: JCAHO, 1994, p 215.

19. *Ibid,* p 703.

20. Burr I: *Statistical Quality Control Methods.* New York: Marcel Dekker, 1976, pp 23–34.

21. Joint Commission on Accreditation of Healthcare Organizations: *Lexikon: Dictionary of Health Care Terms, Organizations, and Acronyms for the Era of Reform,* Oakbrook Terrace, IL: JCAHO, 1994, p 396.

22. Deming WE: *Out of the Crisis.* Cambridge, MA: Massachusetts Institute of Technology, Center for Advanced Engineering Study, 1986.

23. Walton M: *The Deming Management Method.* New York: Perigee Books, Putnam Publishing Group, 1986, p 60.

24. Gitlow H, Gitlow S, Oppenheim A, Oppenheim R: *Tools and Methods for the Improvement of Quality.* Homewood, IL: Irwin, 1989, pp 142–156, 157–213, 214–289.

25. Ibid, p 219.

26. Ibid, p 225.

27. Ibid, pp 190–194.

28. Brassard M, Ritter D: *The Memory Jogger II: A Pocket Guide of Tools for Continuous Improvement and Effective Planning.* Methuen, MA: GOAL/QPC, 1994, p 45.

29. The discussion of logistic regression is excerpted from *Joint Commission Beta II Feedback Report (Cardiovascular Indicators— 1992 [Quarter IV] and 1993 [Quarter I],* 1993.

CHAPTER EIGHT

Determining the Underlying Causes of Undesirable Variation

The major objective of studying variation behavior in clinical performance results is the ability to judge whether a process is in good control. This judgment is critical because it indicates the predictability of future results. Results will be predictable for a process in good control but will be unpredictable for a process that is out of control. The underlying causes of variation should be investigated when a process does not demonstrate a desired level of control.

Underlying causes of variation may be called factors, cause factors, underlying factors, root causes, reasons, underlying reasons, problems, or underlying problems.

Studying Variation Behavior for Performance Improvement Activities

The information contained in variation forms the basis for two broad categories of performance improvement activities: stabilizing an out-of-control process and improving an in-control process.

As described in Chapter Seven, common-cause variation in a series of results requires fundamental changes in the process itself to achieve sustainable change. Variation that is due to special causes requires action to prevent the effects of those causes in the future.

Stabilizing an Out-of-Control Process

The first activity involves taking action on statistical signals of change that are detected in results so that an out-of-control process is brought back to its former condition.[1] The object of stabilizing an out-of-control process is to achieve and maintain a steady state—that is, a steady level of variation around a steady average. Control charts are used to detect special-cause variation. Once a statistical signal of change has been detected in a control chart, the underlying special cause(s) needs to be identified.

Improving an In-Control Process

The second activity concerns processes that are statistically in good control but do not adequately meet customer needs or expectations. As explained in Chapter Seven, good control does not necessarily mean that a given process is adequately meeting customers' expectations or needs. It only means that the process is *consistent*, but it may be consistently mediocre or even consistently bad.[2]

This second activity is intended to identify opportunities for change to the process and its inputs, which are expected to improve all future results. The comparison chart described in Chapter Seven enables interpreters to identify organizational rates that are in good control over time but are inconsistent with the rates of other organizations in the same clinical performance database.

Process performance is most commonly improved by changing the process average indicated by the center line of a control chart. For example, an organization's average for some process is 40% and the process is in good control over time. A comparison chart indicates that the process average for all organizations contributing to the database is 60%, rather than 40%. After investigating the practices leading to the 60% rate, the organization with the 40% average discovers that opportunities exist for improving its own in-control process of care. Process performance improvement for the organization would then consist of moving its process average up toward 60%.

Tools and Methods to Identify Causes of In- and Out-of-Control Process Variation

A large number of tools and methods are available for finding causes of variation. The same tools are used for identifying special causes for out-of-control processes or common causes for in-control processes. These tools and methods include the following: brainstorming, cause-and-effect diagram, checksheet, control chart, flowchart, force field analysis, histogram, nominal group technique, Pareto diagram, process capability, run chart, scatter diagram, and stratification.[1-6]

These techniques for identifying underlying causes of variation can be very helpful when used appropriately. One observer cautions that "too often, a tool for data analysis is used for its own sake, out of the context of systematically building knowledge and taking action for improvement. This may be done in the mistaken belief that the tool is able to lead the user to ask the right questions about the process. Unfortunately no tool is able to provide a rationale for analysis or a substitute for thought."[7]

Dr Kaoru Ishikawa, a Japanese expert on quality control, also warns about the indiscriminate use of quality control tools and techniques. He recalls that in the 1950s the use of certain statistical tools and methods created a number of problems in Japan, including causing fear and dislike of quality control because workers did not understand the methods. He says, "It is true that statistical methods are effective, but we overemphasized their importance. We overeducated people by giving them sophisticated methods where, at that stage, simple methods would have sufficed."[8]

The approach used in this book to identify underlying causes of variation is to focus on five important tools and techniques for understanding causes of variation. They are the flowchart, cause-and-effect diagram, brainstorming, checksheet, and Pareto diagram. There are, however, valuable sources that describe other tools and methods and their various applications.[1–6]

Flowcharting

A *flowchart* is a pictorial summary that shows with symbols and words the steps, sequence, and relationship of the various operations involved in performing a function, such as leadership or patient and family education, or a process, such as ordering a medication.[9] A flowchart enables users to identify the actual and ideal path that any service follows in order to identify deviations. Figures 30 and 31 (see pages 171 and 172) are examples of flowcharts used for functions assessed by the Joint Commission's standards.

Flowcharting a function or a process, as opposed to using written or verbal descriptions, has many advantages.[10] It enables users to understand where they fit into a function or process, how what they do is linked to what others do, and what the end result(s) of a function or process are. Flowcharts help to identify important steps of a function or process, which highlights them for measurement and monitoring. Flowcharting makes it easier to detect problems and opportunities for improvement in a function or a process. Flowcharts provide a record of a function or process. Finally, flowcharts can help people think more clearly as they construct cause-and-effect diagrams, as discussed below.

There are three principles governing the technique of flowcharting:

1. The people who develop a flowchart should be the "owners" of the function or process under study—that is, those individuals directly involved in the activity on a day-to-day basis. For example, owners of the operative and other invasive procedures function would include, at a minimum, physicians (surgeons, anesthetists, emergency physicians, radiologists, pathologists, intensivists), nurses, pharmacists, information management specialists, managers, clerks, and patients. Excluding one or more owners may affect

FIGURE 30 Flowchart of the Leadership Function

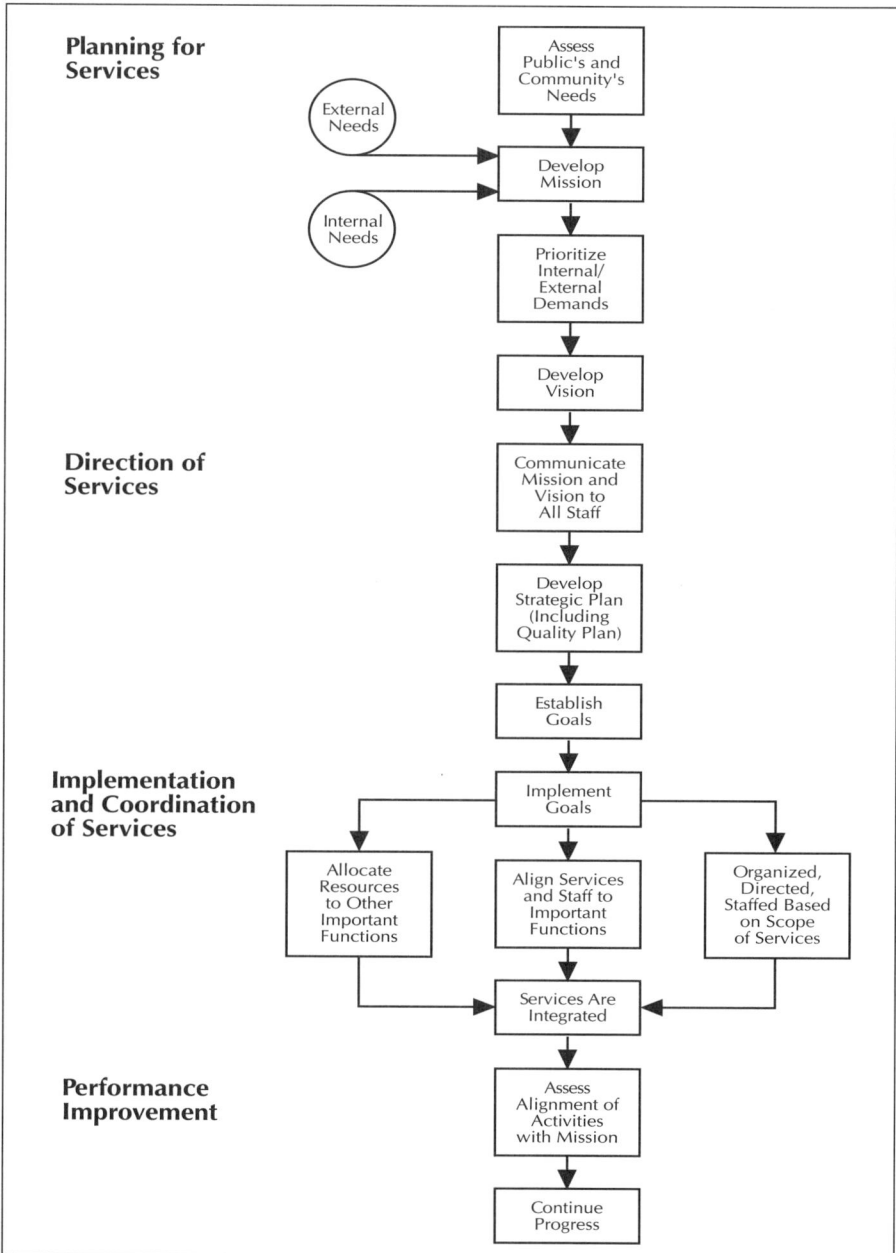

Planning for Services

Assess Public's and Community's Needs

External Needs

Develop Mission

Internal Needs

Prioritize Internal/ External Demands

Develop Vision

Direction of Services

Communicate Mission and Vision to All Staff

Develop Strategic Plan (Including Quality Plan)

Establish Goals

Implementation and Coordination of Services

Implement Goals

Allocate Resources to Other Important Functions

Align Services and Staff to Important Functions

Organized, Directed, Staffed Based on Scope of Services

Services Are Integrated

Performance Improvement

Assess Alignment of Activities with Mission

Continue Progress

This flowchart of the leadership function was developed by the Joint Commission on Accreditation of Healthcare Organizations, Standards Department, 1992. It is currently undergoing testing and is subject to revision.

FIGURE 31 Flowchart of the Operative and Other Invasive Procedures Function

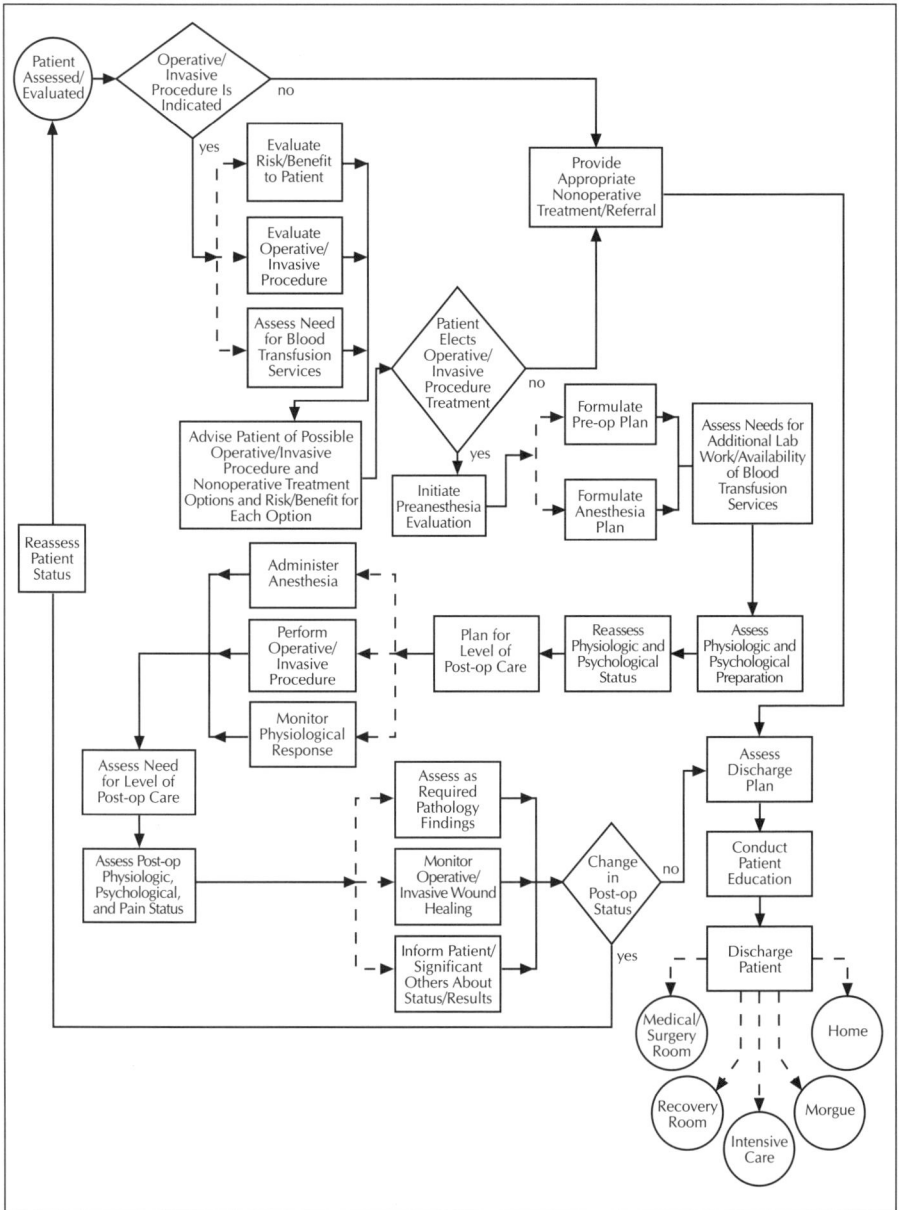

This flowchart of the operative and other invasive procedures function was developed by the Joint Commission on Accreditation of Healthcare Organizations, Standards Department, 1992. It is currently undergoing testing and is subject to revision.

improvement efforts because important input has not been elicited; that input may be key to resolving issues and improving performance and the quality of patient care.

2. The boundaries of the function or process under study should be carefully defined. Boundaries make it easier to establish ownership and highlight connections between a function or process and other functions or processes.

3. Key outcomes (both positive and negative) of a function or process should be identified and measured. Clearly stating the desired goals or outcomes (as well as outcomes to be avoided) of the function or process helps everyone involved with flowcharting work toward the same goals.

Kaoru Ishikawa, Cause-and-Effect Diagrams, and Identifying Causes of Variation

The number of potential underlying causes of variation for any given process is seemingly infinite.[11] Consider, for instance, the number of causes that contribute to the effectiveness of a given procedure (such as coronary artery bypass graft surgery), accuracy in making a specified diagnosis (such as staging breast cancer or diagnosing acute myocardial infarction), timeliness with which a certain treatment is provided (such as laparotomy for hemoperitoneum), or appropriateness with which organizational performance is assessed and improved over time. In each of these instances, most clinicians could rapidly generate a list of 10 or 20 or 30 underlying causes that could be contributing to variation.

A process is nothing more than "a collection of cause factors," according to Ishikawa.[12] With so many potential causes contributing to a given effect—that is, variation—how does one go about identifying the *most important* causes responsible for the variation observed in a series of clinical performance results?

A good place to start is by constructing a *cause-and-effect diagram*, shown in Figure 32 (see page 174). This technique was

FIGURE 32 Example of a Cause-and-Effect Diagram

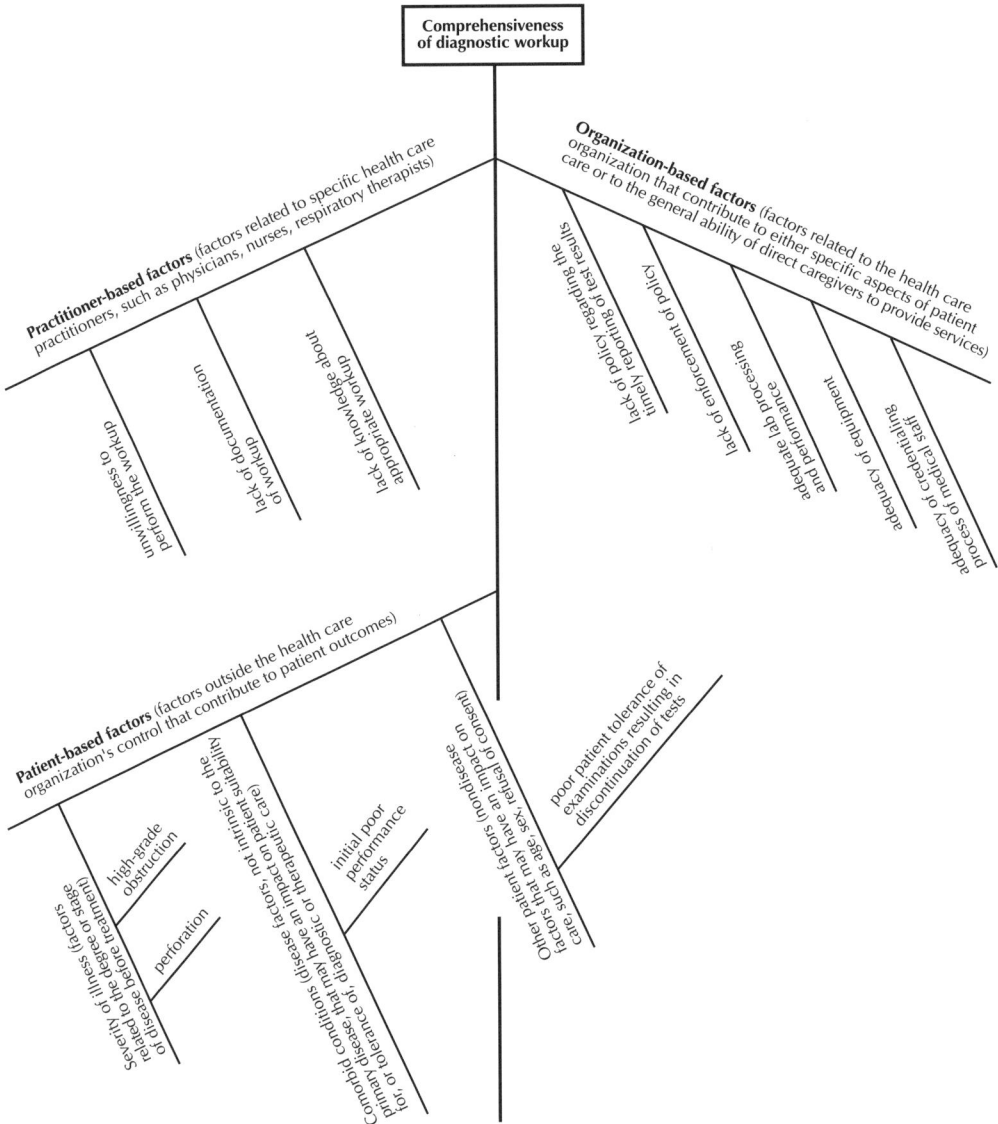

This cause-and-effect diagram outlines the major factors affecting comprehensiveness of diagnostic workups for patients in the indicator group corresponding to the following beta indicator: *Patients with resections of primary colorectal cancer whose preoperative evaluation by a managing physician includes examination of the entire colon, liver function tests, chest x-ray, and carcinoembryonic antigen levels.* This indicator was modified and accepted for inclusion in the IMSystem.

invented by Ishikawa to facilitate the thinking used in process control—that is, "taking hold of the process, which is a collection of cause factors, and building within the process ways of making better products, establishing better goals, and achieving effects." In 1962, Dr Joseph Juran, the American quality control expert, referred to the cause-and-effect diagram as an *Ishikawa diagram* in honor of its inventor. The diagram's shape has also resulted in another nick-name: *fishbone diagram.* All three terms are used with frequency in the literature.

Structure of a Cause-and-Effect Diagram. On the right side of a cause-and-effect diagram, the effect is listed. Examples of effects include prolonged time for surgical intervention for patients with abdominal injuries, or decreased accuracy of diagnosis of acute myocardial infarction.

On the left side of the diagram major causes potentially contrib-uting to the effect are summarized under several branching catego-ries. Ishikawa originally identified five categories to meet his needs (the 5Ms: materials, machines, measurement, man, method) but virtually any categorization can be developed depending on the needs of the interpreters. The underlying causes of the Joint Commission's beta indicators, as described further below, are classi-fied into patient-based, practitioner-based, and organization-based categories.

Constructing a Cause-and-Effect Diagram. The first step in constructing a cause-and-effect diagram is to gather a group of health professionals with expertise in the process or function under-going analysis and ask them to brainstorm to generate the causes needed to construct a cause-and-effect diagram. *Brainstorming* is the process used to elicit large numbers of ideas from a group of people who are encouraged to use their collective thinking power to generate ideas and unrestrained thoughts in a relatively short period.[13]

For instance, Joint Commission Indicator Development Task Forces brainstormed to generate lists of underlying causes that could influence variation in each indicator they developed. The causes were divided into patient-based, practitioner-based, and organization-based categories. The list of underlying causes for each indicator constitutes a section of each indicator's information set as described in Chapters Two and Four. Tables 13–15 (see pages 177–179) are examples of underlying causes developed for a sample of Joint Commission cardiovascular, oncology, and trauma care beta indicators.

Once sufficient ideas have been generated, the actual cause-and-effect diagram is constructed. The problem (effect) is placed in a box on the right side of the diagram. Then on the left side, major cause categories (such as patient-based, practitioner-based, and organization-based) are drawn as branches off of the horizontal trunk in the center.

The brainstormed ideas are then placed in the appropriate major categories (branches). For each cause, one must then ask, "Why does it happen?" Responses to this question are listed as smaller branches off the major causes. Causes that appear repeatedly should be the most basic causes of a problem and are usually selected for further pursuit. Group consensus is also an important means for identifying the most important causes.

Two examples illustrate cause-and-effect diagram construction. The first example involves an organization faced with undesirable variation relating to accuracy in diagnosing acute myocardial infarction (Figure 33; see page 180).* The second example involves an organization faced with undesirable variation for timeliness of surgical intervention for trauma patients with abdominal injuries

---

*The Joint Commission Cardiovascular Care Task Force for Indicator Development developed the following related indicator for beta testing: *Patients admitted for acute myocardial infarction (AMI), rule-out AMI, or unstable angina who have a discharge diagnosis of AMI, subcategorized by admission to an intensive care unit, a monitored bed, or an unmonitored bed.* This indicator was selected in a revised form for inclusion in the IMSystem.

TABLE 13 Underlying Causes for Cardiovascular Care Performance Data*

Indicator (Numerator)
Patients undergoing attempted or completed percutaneous transluminal coronary angioplasty (PTCA) during which any lesion attempted is not dilated.

Underlying Factors
Factors not included in the indicator that may account for significant indicator rates or indicator activity.

A. Patient-based factors (factors outside the health care organization's control that contribute to patient outcomes)

   1. Severity of illness (factors related to the degree or stage of disease before treatment)

      a. left ventricular dysfunction

      b. multivessel disease

      c. preprocedure total chronic occlusion

      d. calcified lesion

      e. history of failed PTCAs

      f. "complex lesion"

   2. Comorbid conditions (disease factors, not intrinsic to the primary disease, that may have an impact on patient suitability for, or tolerance of, diagnostic or therapeutic care)

      a. diabetes mellitus

      b. peripheral vascular disease

   3. Other patient factors (nondisease factors that may have an impact on care, for example, age, sex, refusal of consent)

      a. age greater that 70

      b. small coronary vessels

B. Nonpatient-based factors

   1. Practitioner-based factors (factors related to specific health care practitioners, such as physicians, nurses, respiratory therapists)

      a. inadequate training and experience of physician

      b. schedule overload

      c. inappropriate use of equipment

      d. inadequate selection of catheters

   2. Organization-based factors (factors related to the health care organization that contribute to either specific aspects of patient care or to the general ability of direct caregivers to provide services)

      a. inadequate maintenance of equipment

      b. schedule overload

      c. inadequate credentialing process

      d. inadequate or inappropriate training of personnel

*The Joint Commission Cardiovascular Care Task Force for Indicator Development developed the indicator and its underlying causes.

TABLE 14 Underlying Causes for Oncology Care Performance Data*

Indicator (Numerator)

Patients with American Joint Committee on Cancer Stage II or III primary rectal cancer with documentation of referral to, or treatment by, a radiation or medical oncologist.

Underlying Factors

Factors not included in the indicator that may account for significant indicator rates or indicator activity.

A. Patient-based factors (factors outside the health care organization's control that contribute to patient outcomes)

1. Severity of illness (factors related to the degree or stage of disease before treatment)
   a. advanced disease
   b. infectious complications
2. Comorbid conditions (disease factors, not intrinsic to the primary disease, that may have an impact on patient suitability for, or tolerance of, diagnostic or therapeutic care)
   a. initial poor performance status
   b. medical contraindications to radiation therapy, for example, autoimmune disease with radiation sensitivity
3. Other patient factors (nondisease factors that may have an impact on care, for example, age, sex, refusal of consent)
   a. patient refusal of radiation therapy
   b. patient is subject in hospital Institutional Review Board–approved research protocol not using radiation therapy

B. Nonpatient-based factors

1. Practitioner-based factors
   a. lack of knowledge about the value of radiotherapy for Stage II disease
   b. inadequate interdisciplinary treatment planning
   c. lack of documentation of referral/consultation
   d. unwillingness to consider radiation therapy in management program
2. Organization-based factors (factors related to the health care organization that contribute to either specific aspects of patient care or to the general ability of direct caregivers to provide services)
   a. lack of system for referral to radiation therapy

*The Joint Commission Oncology Care Task Force for Indicator Development developed the indicator and its underlying causes.

TABLE 15 Underlying Causes for Trauma Care Performance Data*

Indicator (Numerator)
Intrahospital mortality of trauma patients with one or more of the following conditions who did not undergo a procedure for the condition: tension pneumothorax, hemoperitoneum, hemothoraces, ruptured aorta, pericardial tamponade, and epidural or subdural hemorrhage.

Underlying Factors
Factors not included in the indicator that may account for significant indicator rates or indicator activity.

A. Patient-based factors (factors outside the health care organization's control that contribute to patient outcomes)
    1. Severity of illness (factors related to the degree or stage of disease before treatment)
        a. injury severity
        b. initial physiologic measurements
        c. multiple-system injury
    2. Comorbid conditions (disease factors, not intrinsic to the primary disease, that may have an impact on patient suitability for, or tolerance of, diagnostic or therapeutic care)
        a. preexisting disease
    3. Other patient factors (nondisease factors that may have an impact on care, for example, age, sex, refusal of consent)
        a. geographic distance between initial hospital and hospital receiving patient in transfer
        b. mode of ambulance transport (air versus ground)
        c. age

B. Nonpatient-based factors
    1. Practitioner-based factors (factors related to specific health care practitioners, such as physicians, nurses, respiratory therapists)
        a. failure of physician to diagnose condition
        b. untimely assessment of patient's condition by physician
        c. ineffective stabilization by physician
        d. inappropriate decision by physician to transfer/not transfer patient
    2. Organization-based factors (factors related to the health care organization that contribute to either specific aspects of patient care or to the general ability of direct caregivers to provide services)
        a. unavailability of resources at initial hospital, such as operating room, intensive care unit beds, specialty services, specialty equipment
        b. hospital's financial commitment to trauma care

*The Joint Commission Trauma Care Task Force for Indicator Development developed the indicator and its underlying causes.

FIGURE 33 Cause-and-Effect Diagram for Cardiovascular Care Performance Data

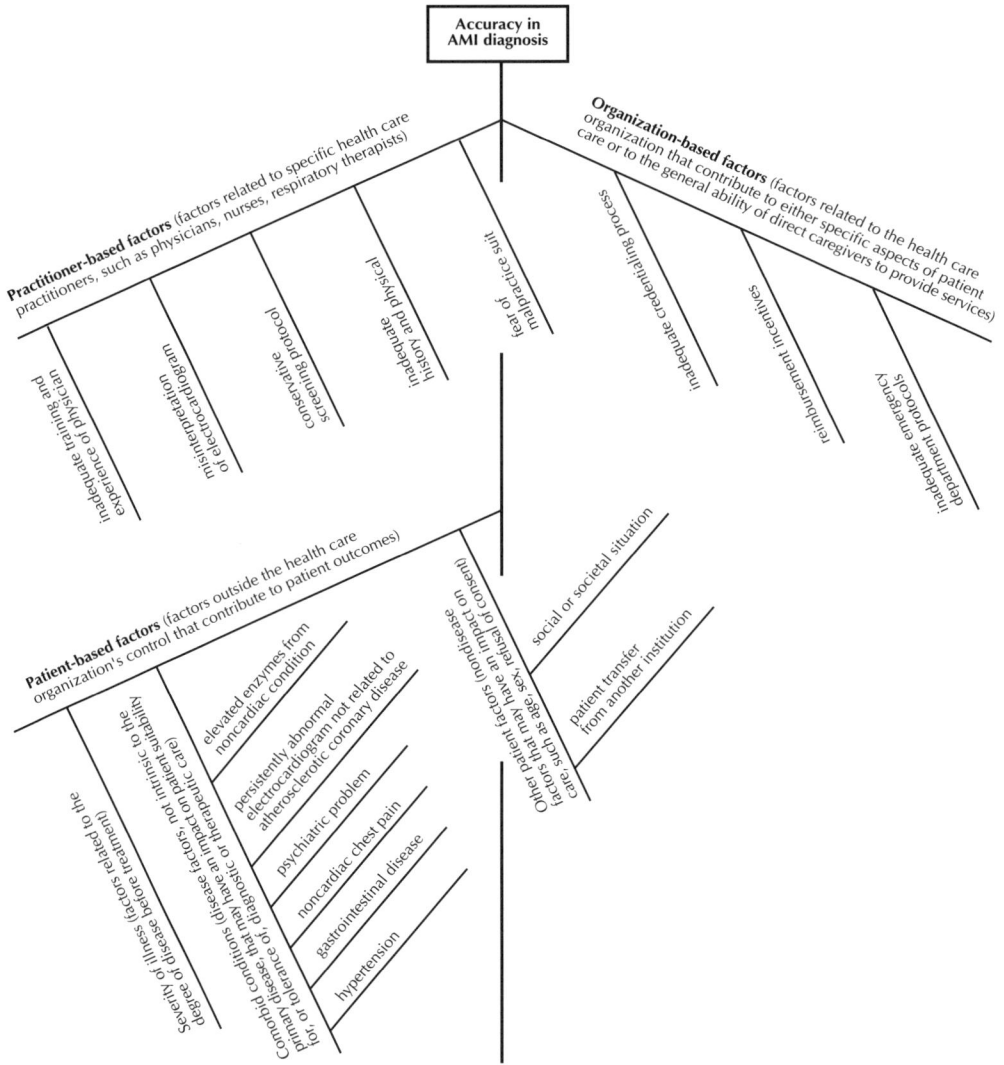

This cause-and-effect diagram generated underlying causes for variation in accurately diagnosing acute myocardial infarction. The Joint Commission Cardiovascular Care Task Force for Indicator Development developed the following related indicator and underlying causes for beta testing: *Patients admitted for acute myocardial infarction (AMI), rule-out AMI, or unstable angina who have a discharge diagnosis of AMI, subcategorized by admission to an intensive care unit, a monitored bed, or an unmonitored bed.* This indicator was selected in a revised form for inclusion in the IMSystem.

FIGURE 34 Cause-and-Effect Diagram for Trauma Care Performance Data

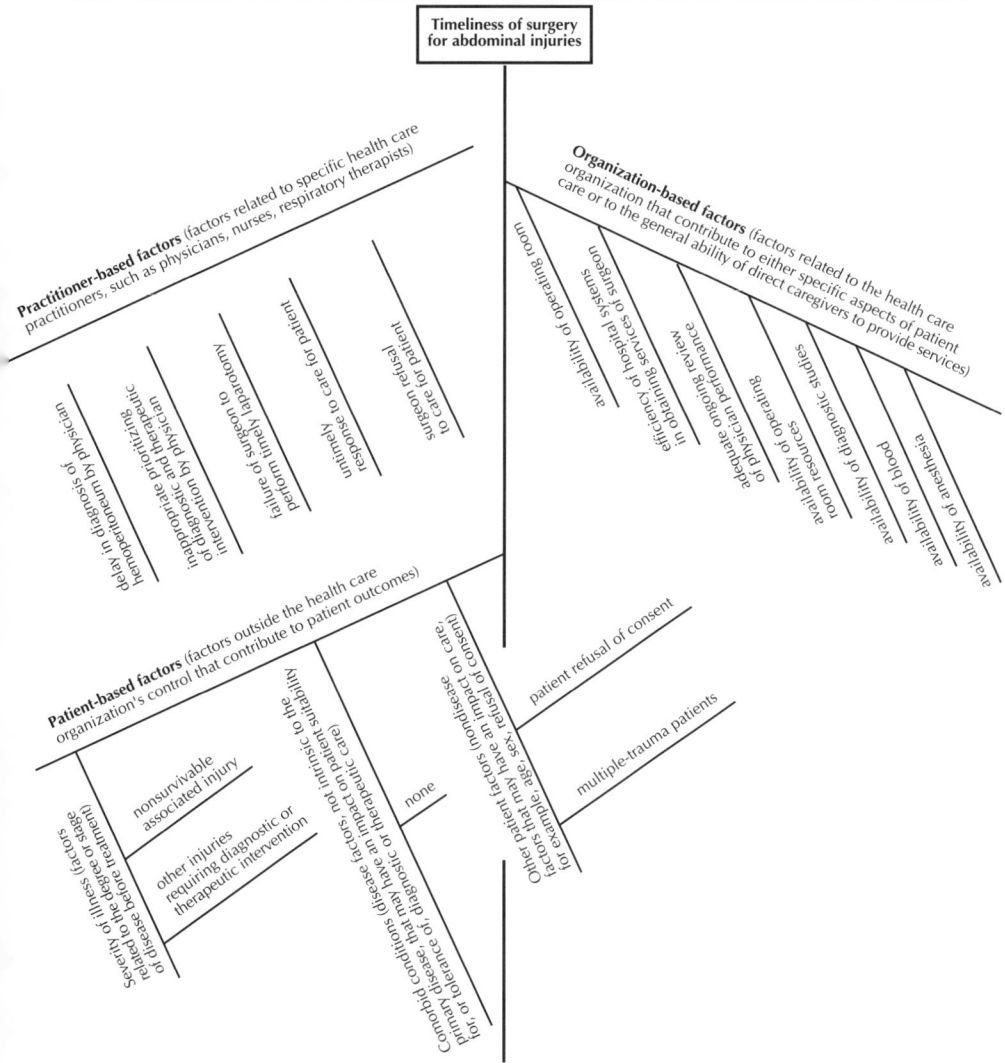

This cause-and-effect diagram generated underlying causes for variation in timeliness of surgery for abdominal injuries. The Joint Commission Trauma Care Task Force for Indicator Development developed the following related indicator and underlying causes for beta testing: *Trauma patients with diagnosis of laceration of liver or spleen requiring surgery undergoing laparotomy greater than two hours after emergency department arrival, subcategorized by pediatric or adult patients.* This indicator was selected in a revised form for inclusion in the IMSystem.

(Figure 34; see page 181).* In each case, underlying causes are divided into patient-based, practitioner-based, and organization-based, which form the major branches off the horizontal trunk of the cause-and-effect diagram.

Advantages and Limitations of Cause-and-Effect Diagrams. There are several advantages of constructing a cause-and-effect diagram to further understand the causes of variation in results. First, a cause-and-effect diagram untangles and orders the web of causes that may contribute to observed variation. Second, it captures the knowledge of a team of people and puts it into a form that is easily communicated and understood. Third, it can help a team decide where to focus its investigative efforts to improve a process or system. Fourth, it is relatively easy to remember as the first step in understanding the causes of variation because of its name.

The limitations of a cause-and-effect diagram relate to its inability to capture the complexity of many processes. For instance, it suggests direct linear relationships and does not imply interdependencies or interactions. Inadequate training and experience of a physician, a practitioner-based cause, may be identified as an underlying cause of unacceptable variation in accurately diagnosing acute myocardial infarction. This cause may be closely linked to an inadequate credentialing or proctoring process, which is an organization-based cause. A cause-and-effect diagram will not describe this linkage.

Use of a Cause-and-Effect Diagram. The cause-and-effect diagram is used to generate the underlying causes of variation. These causes are further analyzed according to the Pareto principle.

---

* The Joint Commission Trauma Care Task Force for Indicator Development developed the following related indicator for beta testing: *Trauma patients with diagnosis of laceration of liver or spleen requiring surgery undergoing laparotomy greater than two hours after emergency department arrival, subcategorized by pediatric or adult patients.* This indicator was selected in a revised form for inclusion in the IMSystem.

Vilfredo Pareto, Pareto Diagrams, and the "Vital Few"

The number of underlying causes for undesirable variation in data can be very large. Even if one wished to address and control every cause, the task would be economically unfeasible. How, then, does an organization decide what causes to work on and in what order?

Vilfredo Pareto (1848–1923) was an Italian economist and sociologist who developed a solution to this conundrum. He identified what he called the "vital few" to help direct resources and attention to areas where they do the most good.[14] The "vital few" is contrasted with the "trivial many," which are the remaining causes in Pareto analysis after the "vital few" have been identified.

The Pareto principle is the basis for the "80-20 rule" articulated by time-management specialist Alan Laeklin.[14] This rule says that approximately 80% of the value comes from 20% of the elements. For instance, 80% of a problem, such as prolonged time in surgical intervention for abdominal injuries, would come from 20% of the causes comprising the process of patient care. Pareto analysis involves determining which few causes of a process are vital and taking action to address these causes, rather than the innumerable other incidental causes that may be contributing to the undesirable variation.

Although Pareto analysis is commonly thought of as a problem-solving tool, it really helps determine *what* problems to solve, rather than *how* to solve them.[14] The process of arranging, classifying, and tabulating the data helps determine the most important causes that require attention from an organization.

Structure of a Pareto Diagram. A Pareto diagram (also called a Pareto chart) is a simple bar chart with the vertical bars representing the frequency of each underlying cause, arranged in descending order along a horizontal axis (see Figure 35, page 184). The principle behind a Pareto diagram is that an organization gains more by working on the tallest bar than working on the shorter bars.

Constructing a Pareto Diagram. There are several important steps in constructing a Pareto diagram. For example, an organization

FIGURE 35 Example of Pareto Diagram

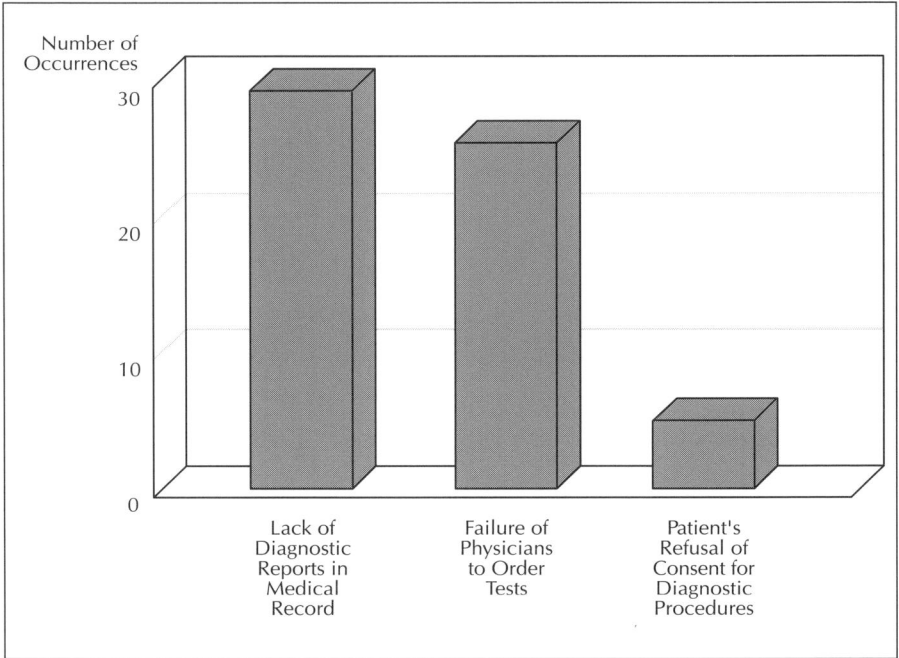

A Pareto diagram lists, in descending order, the "vital few" underlying causes of variation. The Joint Commission Cardiovascular Care Task Force for Indicator Development developed the following related indicator and underlying causes for beta testing: *Patients with principal discharge diagnosis of congestive heart failure (CHF) with documented etiology and chest x-ray substantiation of CHF.* This indicator was selected in a revised form for inclusion in the IMSystem.

has monitored timeliness of surgical intervention for abdominal injuries over time. Astute interpreters have determined that the process is in good control for the organization, but that the average minutes fall outside the prediction interval on the indicator's comparison chart (meaning the process is operating at a significantly different level from other organizations contributing to the performance database). This observation leads the interpreters to ask why. The organization constructs the cause-and-effect diagram shown in Figure 34 and is now ready to construct a Pareto diagram.

The following steps are recommended by Ishikawa and other quality control experts for constructing a Pareto diagram.[14] *First, establish the categories for the data undergoing analysis.* In the timeliness of surgical intervention example in Figure 34, the categories include all the causes relating to practitioner-based factors (for example, surgeon refusal to care for patient), organization-based factors (for example, availability of anesthesia), and patient-based factors (for example, patient refusal of consent for surgery). These potential causes can be tabulated for further study, as shown in Table 16 (see page 186).

If the number of causes is very large, brainstorming and consensus building can be used to narrow the possibilities to, say, the 10 most likely possibilities. Pareto's dictum states that the number of truly important causes that sharply influence results is limited. In searching for these important causes, it is important that all people who are familiar with a particular process be consulted. They must be able to discuss the process openly and frankly. It would be inappropriate, for example, for an organization to exclude certain experts because they were not liked or their views about the issue were not welcome. Table 17 (see page 187) shows how a cross-departmental and cross-disciplinary trauma team used brainstorming to narrow the list to eight potential causes.

Second, collect additional data during a specified time period for each of the categories to determine how often a given cause contributes to the undesirable variation observed in the data. In the timeliness of surgical intervention example, the team chose a one-month period to collect additional data for each of the cause categories. Representatives of the team concurrently reviewed the emergency department record, operating room record, and other source documents for each trauma patient with abdominal injuries whose transfer to the operating room from the emergency department was greater than 60 minutes after arrival to the emergency department. They also interviewed numerous hospital staff with knowledge about the process. The results of their data collection was

TABLE 16 Tabulated Causes for Delayed Surgery for Abdominal Injuries*

- Other injuries requiring diagnostic or therapeutic intervention
- Nonsurvivable associated injury
- Availability of operating room
- Efficiency of hospital systems in obtaining services of surgeon
- Adequacy of ongoing review of physician performance
- Availability of operating room resources
- Availability of diagnostic studies
- Patient refusal of consent
- Multiple-trauma patients
- Delay in diagnosis of hemoperitoneum by physician
- Inappropriate prioritizing of diagnostic and therapeutic intervention by physician
- Failure of surgeon to perform timely laparotomy
- Untimely response to care for patient
- Surgeon refusal to care for patient
- Availability of blood
- Availability of anesthesia

*The Joint Commission Trauma Care Task Force for Indicator Development developed the following related indicator and underlying causes for beta testing: *Trauma patients with diagnosis of laceration of liver or spleen requiring surgery undergoing laparotomy greater than two hours after emergency department arrival, subcategorized by pediatric or adult patients.* This indicator was selected in a revised form for inclusion in the IMSystem.

a checksheet that recorded the sources of delay in surgical intervention for abdominal injuries (see Figure 36, page 188).

A *checksheet* is simply a data collection form that summarizes counts for individual cause categories. It is used to answer the question, "How often are certain events happening?" It is key to translating opinions into facts.[15] In the current example, for

TABLE 17 Eight Most Important Causes for Delayed Surgery for Abdominal Injuries

- Availability of operating room
- Availability of diagnostic studies
- Efficiency of hospital systems in obtaining services of surgeon
- Delay in diagnosis of hemoperitoneum by physician
- Failure of surgeon to perform timely laparotomy
- Untimely response to care for patient
- Surgeon refusal to care for patient
- Availability of anesthesia

instance, one expert involved in studying variation may be quite certain that the variation is due to the unavailability of operating rooms. Another expert may be certain that it is due to delayed responses of surgeons to evaluate newly arrived trauma patients in the emergency department. A third expert may believe that the variation is due to lack of timely diagnostic imaging procedures (x-rays or computerized axial tomography) because the response by diagnostic imaging personnel (technicians, radiologists) is slow. Actual counts of each category provide the "facts" that can buttress or refute expert opinions. It is often helpful to translate counts into relative frequencies to gain a clearer understanding of how much individual causes are contributing to the problem (see Figure 37, page 189).

Third, use the checksheet data (counts or relative frequencies) to construct a Pareto diagram. Horizontal and vertical axes are drawn. The vertical axis is marked with units for number of occurrences (for counts) or percentages (for relative frequencies). The horizontal axis is marked with individual cause categories. The most frequently occurring cause category is always placed first on the far left, followed by the next most frequent cause category, and so on to the right.

FIGURE 36 Checksheet for Sources of Delay in Surgical Intervention for Abdominal Injuries

Cause Category	Number of Occurrences	
Unavailability of operating room	ЖЖ ЖЖ ΙΙ	12
Unavailability of diagnostic studies	ЖЖ ЖЖ ЖЖ Ι	16
Inefficiency of hospital systems in obtaining services of surgeon	ΙΙ	2
Delay in diagnosing hemoperitoneum by physician	ЖЖ ΙΙΙ	8
Failure of surgeon to perform timely laparotomy	ЖЖ Ι	6
Untimely response to care for patient	ΙΙΙ	3
Surgeon's refusal to care for patient	Ι	1
Unavailability of anesthesia	ЖЖ ЖЖ ΙΙ	12
Total		60

The second step in constructing a Pareto diagram is collecting additional data to determine how often each cause contributes to the undesirable variation.

Figure 38 (see page 190) is a Pareto diagram for the timeliness of surgical intervention example. Approximately 80% of the problem comes from approximately 20% of the causes—that is, one of the six categories of causes (16%) constitutes 80% of the problem. This agrees with the "80-20 rule" described earlier.

FIGURE 37 Frequency Table for Sources of Delay in Surgical Intervention for Abdominal Injuries

Cause Category	Number of Occurrences	Relative Frequency
Unavailability of operating room	12	20%
Unavailability of diagnostic studies	16	27%
Inefficiency of hospital systems in obtaining services of surgeon	2	3%
Delay in diagnosing hemoperitoneum by physician	8	13%
Failure of surgeon to perform timely laparotomy	6	10%
Untimely response to care for patient	3	5%
Surgeon's refusal to care for patient	1	2%
Unavailability of anesthesia	12	20%
Total	60	100%

Relative frequencies for each cause give a clearer picture of how much each cause is contributing to the problem.

In Figure 39 (see page 191), however, 66% of the causes constitute 80% of the problem—that is, four of the six categories of causes (66%) contribute to 80% of the problem. This example ignores the 80-20 rule. Thus, although the 80-20 breakdown is a frequent Pareto occurrence, it is neither a rule nor a requirement.

FIGURE 38 Pareto Diagram for Sources of Delay in Surgical Intervention for Abdominal Injuries: 80-20 Rule

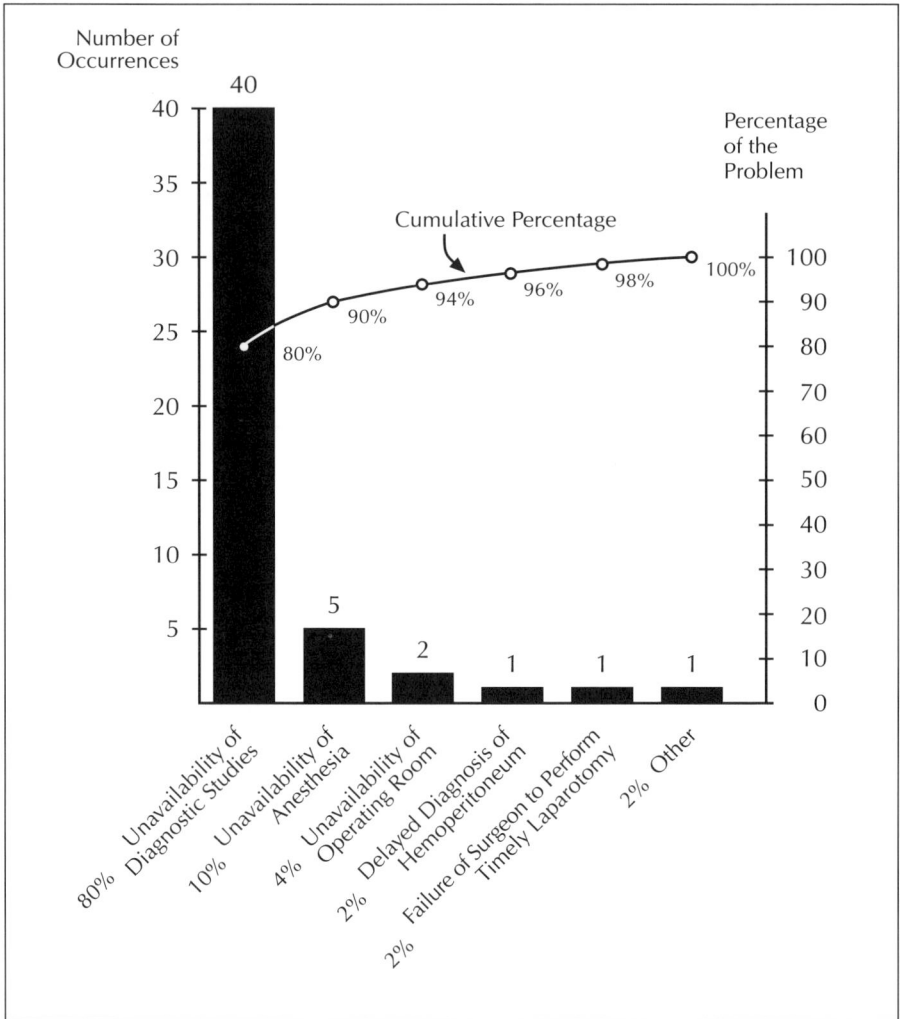

This Pareto diagram illustrates the "80-20" rule—that 80% of the problem lies in 20% of the causes.

Applications of Pareto Diagrams. The main purpose of constructing a Pareto diagram is to focus attention on which major problem or problems a team should concentrate its improvement efforts. In the timeliness of surgical intervention example, the un-availability of diagnostic studies (namely, diagnostic imaging and

FIGURE 39 Pareto Diagram for Sources of Delay in Surgical Intervention for Abdominal Injuries

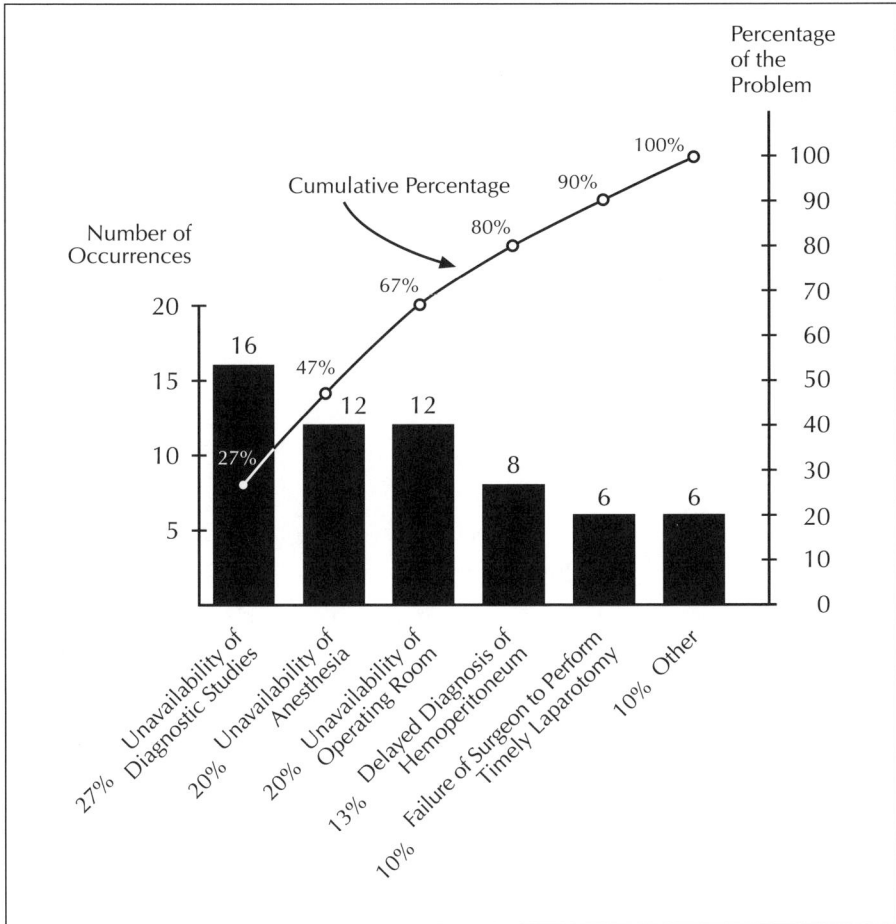

This Pareto diagram breaks the "80-20 rule"; instead, 66% of the causes constitute 80% of the problem.

laboratory studies) was the main cause of delays in getting patients with abdominal injuries to the operating room in a timely manner. Operating room and anesthesia unavailability ranked second and third. These "vital few" causes form the basis for improvement efforts. Clearly, the organization has a challenging agenda.

Pareto diagrams also can be very helpful in determining whether improvement efforts are producing desired results. If improvement has occurred, the order of the items on the horizontal axis changes. In the before-improvement Pareto diagram (see Figure 38) for the timeliness of surgical intervention example, the major cause of delays was unavailability of diagnostic studies. After improvements to the process are made, the major cause should become the least frequent cause if the improvements are producing their intended effect. The organization would next address the unavailability of operating rooms and anesthesia, which are now ranked first and second. Using a Pareto diagram as an improvement gauge is powerful because the vertical bars are simple and easy for people to comprehend. Workers can take heart as each towering bar is toppled, an indication that the process is improving.

Summary Observations

Understanding the causes of variation in a series of clinical performance results is the final task of the interpretive process. It lays out the causes of variation and prioritizes the order in which the causes should be addressed. It also provides a gauge for determining whether changes that have been implemented are producing the desired effect. There are several important points about underlying causes in this chapter:

1. The number of potential causes for any given process is infinite.

2. A process is a collection of cause factors.

3. A flowchart is a pictorial summary that shows with symbols and words the steps, sequence, and relationship of the various operations involved in performing a function or process.

4. A cause-and-effect diagram enables interpreters to identify the causes responsible for the variation observed in clinical performance results.

5. Brainstorming elicits large numbers of ideas from a group that is encouraged to use its collective thinking power to generate ideas and unrestrained thoughts in a relatively short period. Brainstorming is often used to generate the underlying causes for a cause-and-effect diagram.

6. Pareto analysis involves determining which few causes of a process are vital and taking action to address these causes, rather than the innumerable other incidental causes that may be contributing to the undesirable variation.

7. The "80-20 rule," based on the Pareto principle, says that approximately 80% of the value comes from 20% of the elements. For instance, 80% of a problem, such as delay in surgical intervention for abdominal injuries, comes from 20% of the causes constituting the process of patient care.

8. A checksheet is a data collection form that summarizes counts for individual cause categories. It is used to answer the question, "How often are certain events happening?" and is key to translating opinions into facts. It is used in constructing a Pareto diagram.

9. The main purpose of constructing a Pareto diagram is to focus attention on which major problem or problems ("vital few") an organization should concentrate its improvement efforts. A Pareto diagram can also determine whether improvement efforts are producing desired results.

References

1.   Bounds G, Yorks L, Adams M, et al: *Beyond Total Quality Management: Toward the Emerging Paradigm.* New York: McGraw-Hill, 1994, p 392.

2.   Brassard M, Ritter D: *The Memory Jogger II: A Pocket Guide of Tools for Continuous Improvement and Effective Planning.* Methuen, MA: GOAL/QPC, 1994, p 52.

3.   Gitlow H, Gitlow S, Oppenheim A, et al: *Tools and Methods for the Improvement of Quality.* Homewood, IL: Irwin, 1989.

4.   Joint Commission on Accreditation of Healthcare Organizations: *Using Quality Improvement Tools in a Health Care Setting.* Oakbrook Terrace, IL: JCAHO, 1992.

5.   Joint Commission on Accreditation of Healthcare Organizations: *Framework for Improving Performance.* Oakbrook Terrace, IL: JCAHO, 1992, pp 83–111.

6. Ishikawa K (David Lu, trans): *What Is Total Quality Control? The Japanese Way*. Englewood Cliffs, NJ: Prentice-Hall, 1985.

7. Bounds G, Yorks L, Adams M, et al: *Beyond Total Quality Management: Toward the Emerging Paradigm*. New York: McGraw-Hill, 1994, p 393.

8. Ishikawa K (David Lu, trans): *What Is Total Quality Control? The Japanese Way*. Englewood Cliffs, NJ: Prentice-Hall, 1985, pp 18–19.

9. Joint Commission on Accreditation of Healthcare Organizations: *Lexikon: Dictionary of Health Care Terms, Organizations, and Acronyms for the Era of Reform*. Oakbrook Terrace, IL: JCAHO, 1994, p 315.

10. Gitlow H, Gitlow S, Oppenheim A, et al: *Tools and Methods for the Improvement of Quality*. Homewood, IL: Irwin, 1989, p 46.

11. Ishikawa K (David Lu, trans): *What Is Total Quality Control? The Japanese Way*. Englewood Cliffs, NJ: Prentice-Hall, 1985, p 64.

12. Ibid, p 63.

13. Joint Commission on Accreditation of Healthcare Organizations: *Lexikon: Dictionary of Health Care Terms, Organizations, and Acronyms for the Era of Reform*. Oakbrook Terrace, IL: JCAHO, 1994, p 149.

14. Gitlow H, Gitlow S, Oppenheim A, et al: *Tools and Methods for the Improvement of Quality*. Homewood, IL: Irwin, 1989, pp 389–390.

15. Joint Commission on Accreditation of Healthcare Organizations: *Lexikon: Dictionary of Health Care Terms, Organizations, and Acronyms for the Era of Reform*. Oakbrook Terrace, IL: JCAHO, 1994, p 174.

APPENDIX A

Joint Commission's Beta-Tested Indicators

ANESTHESIA CARE Indicators for Beta Testing

AN-1

Indicator (Numerator): Patients developing a CNS complication during or within two postprocedure days of procedures involving anesthesia administration, subcategorized by ASA-PS class, patient age, and CNS versus non-CNS related procedures.

AN-2

Indicator (Numerator): Patients developing a peripheral neurologic deficit during or within two postprocedure days of procedures involving anesthesia administration.

AN-3

Indicator (Numerator): Patients developing an acute myocardial infarction during or within two postprocedure days of procedures involving anesthesia administration, subcategorized by ASA-PS class, patient age, and cardiac versus noncardiac procedures.

AN-4

Indicator (Numerator): Patients with a cardiac arrest during or within one postprocedure day of procedures involving anesthesia administration, excluding patients with required intraoperative cardiac arrest, subcategorized by ASA-PS class, patient age, and cardiac vs noncardiac procedures.

AN-5

Indicator (Numerator): Patients with unplanned respiratory arrest during or within one postprocedure day involving anesthesia administration.

AN-6

Indicator (Numerator): Death of patients during or within two postprocedure days of procedures involving anesthesia administration, subcategorized by class and patient age.

AN-7

Indicator (Numerator): Unplanned admission of patients to the hospital within one postprocedure day following outpatient procedures involving anesthesia administration.

AN-8

Indicator (Numerator): Unplanned admission of patients to an intensive care unit within one postprocedure day of procedures involving anesthesia administration and with ICU stay greater than one day.

OBSTETRICAL CARE Indicators for Beta Testing

OB-1

Indicator (Numerator): Patients with primary cesarean section for failure to progress.

OB-2

Indicator (Numerator): Patients with attempted vaginal birth after cesarean section (VBAC), subcategorized by success or failure.

OB-3

Indicator (Numerator): Patients with excessive maternal blood loss defined by intrapartum and/or postpartum red blood cell transfusion or a low post-delivery hematocrit or hemoglobin (Hct<22%, Hgb<7 gms) or a significant pre- to post-delivery decrease in hematocrit (>11%) or hemoglobin (>3.5 gms) excluding patients with abruptio placenta or placenta previa.

OB-4

Indicator (Numerator): Patients with diagnosis of eclampsia.

OB-5

Indicator (Numerator): The delivery of infants weighing less than 2,500 grams following either induction of labor or repeat cesarean section without medical indications.

OB-6

Indicator (Numerator): Term infants admitted to an NICU within one day of delivery and with NICU stay greater than one day excluding admission for major congenital anomalies.

OB-7

Indicator (Numerator): Neonates with an Apgar score of 3 or less at 5 minutes and a birthweight greater than 1,500 grams.

OB-8

Indicator (Numerator): Neonates with a discharge diagnosis of significant birth trauma.

OB-9

Indicator (Numerator): Term infants with a diagnosis of hypoxic encephalopathy or clinically apparent seizure prior to discharge from the hospital of birth excluding newborns with a diagnosis of fetal alcohol syndrome, and other drug reactions and withdrawal syndromes.

OB-10

Indicator (Numerator): Deaths of infants weighing 500 grams or more subcategorized by intrahospital neonatal deaths, total stillborns, and intrapartum stillborns.

ONCOLOGY Indicators for Beta Testing

Oncology Indicator Patient Population: Inpatients admitted for initial diagnosis and/or treatment of primary lung, colon, rectal, or female breast cancer.

ON-1

Indicator Focus: Availability of data for diagnosis and staging. **Indicator (Numerator):** Surgical pathology consultation reports (pathology reports) containing histological type, tumor size, status of margins, appropriate lymph node examination, assessment of invasion or extension as indicated, and AJCC/pTN classification for patients with resection for primary cancer of the lung, colon/rectum, or female breast.

ON-2

Indicator Focus: Use of staging by managing physicians. **Indicator (Numerator):** Patients undergoing treatment for primary cancer of the lung, colon/rectum, or female breast with AJCC stage of tumor designated by a managing physician.

ON-3

Indicator Focus: Effectiveness of cancer treatment. **Indicator (Numerator):** Survival of patients with primary cancer of the lung, colon/rectum, or female breast by stage and histologic type.

ON-4

Indicator Focus: Use of tests critical to diagnosis, prognosis, and clinical management. **Indicator (Numerator):** Female patients with invasive primary breast cancer undergoing initial biopsy or resection of a tumor larger than one centimeter in greatest dimension who have presence of estrogen receptor diagnostic analysis results in medical record.

ON-5

Indicator Focus: Use of multimodal therapy in treatment and follow-up. **Indicator (Numerator):** Female patients with AJCC Stage II pathologic lymph node positive primary invasive breast cancer treated with systemic adjuvant therapy.

ON-6

Indicator Focus: Effectiveness of preoperative diagnosis and staging. **Indicator (Numerator):** Patients with non-small cell primary lung cancer undergoing thoracotomy with complete surgical resection of tumor.

ON-7

Indicator Focus: Specific clinical events as a means of assessing multiple aspects of surgical care for lung cancers. **Indicator (Numerator):** Patients undergoing pulmonary resection for primary lung cancer with postoperative complication of empyema, bronchopleural fistula, reoperation for postoperative bleeding, mechanical ventilation greater than 5 days postop, or intrahospital death.

ON-8

Indicator Focus: Comprehensiveness of diagnostic workup. **Indicator (Numerator):** Patients with resection of primary colorectal cancer whose preoperative evaluation by a managing physician includes examination of the entire colon, liver function tests, chest x-ray, and carcinoembryonic antigen (CEA) levels.

ON-9

Indicator Focus: Documentation of staging, prognosis, and surgical treatment. **Indicator (Numerator):** Patients with resection of primary colorectal cancer whose operative reports include location of primary tumor, local extent of disease, extent of resection, and assessment of residual abdominal disease.

ON-10

Indicator Focus: Use of treatment approaches that impact on quality of life. **Indicator (Numerator):** Patients with primary rectal cancer undergoing abdominoperineal resections with 6 cm or more of free distal surgical margin present on specimen, as documented in surgical pathology gross description.

ON-11

Indicator Focus: Interdisciplinary treatment and follow-up. **Indicator (Numerator):** Patients with AJCC Stage II or III primary rectal cancer with documentation of referral to or treatment by a radiation or medical oncologist.

CARDIOVASCULAR Indicators for Beta Testing

Cardiovascular Indicator Patient Population: The cardiovascular indicators draw from four populations described below: coronary artery bypass grafts (CABG), percutaneous transluminal coronary angioplasty (PTCA), acute myocardial infarction (MI), and congestive heart failure (CHF).

CABG Patient Population: Patients undergoing coronary artery bypass grafts (CABG) excluding those with other cardiac or peripheral vascular surgical procedures performed at the time of the CABG (eg, valve replacement).

CV-1

Indicator Focus: Intrahospital mortality as a means of assessing multiple aspects of CABG care. **Indicator (Numerator):** Intrahospital mortality of patients undergoing isolated coronary artery bypass graft (CABG) procedures, subcategorized by initial or subsequent CABG procedures, by emergent or nonemergent clinical status, and by postoperative day and intrahospital location of death.

CV-2

Indicator Focus: Extended postoperative stay as a means of assessing multiple aspects of CABG care. **Indicator (Numerator):** Patients with prolonged postoperative stay for isolated coronary artery bypass graft (CABG) procedures, subcategorized by initial or subsequent CABG procedures, by emergent or nonemergent procedures, and by the use or nonuse of a circulatory support device.

PTCA Patient Population: Patients for whom a percutaneous transluminal coronary angioplasty (PTCA) procedure is initiated, regardless of whether or not a lesion is crossed or dilated.

CV-3

Indicator Focus: Intrahospital mortality as a means of assessing multiple aspects of PTCA care. **Indicator (Numerator):**

Intrahospital mortality of patients following percutaneous transluminal coronary angioplasty (PTCA), subcategorized by emergent or nonemergent clinical status and by postprocedure day and intrahospital location of death.

CV-4

Indicator Focus: Specific clinical events as a means of assessing multiple aspects of PTCA care. **Indicator (Numerator):** Patients undergoing nonemergent percutaneous transluminal coronary angioplasty (PTCA) with subsequent occurrence of either an acute myocardial infarction (MI) or coronary artery bypass graft (CABG) procedure within the same hospitalization.

CV-5

Indicator Focus: Effectiveness of PTCA. **Indicator (Numerator):** Patients undergoing attempted or completed percutaneous transluminal coronary angioplasty (PTCA) during which any lesion attempted is not dilated.

MI Patient Population: Patients with a principal diagnosis of acute myocardial infarction (MI) either upon hospital discharge, emergency department (ED) transfer to another acute care facility, or death in the emergency department (ED), and patients who are admitted for an acute MI or to rule out an acute MI.

CV-6

Indicator Focus: Intrahospital mortality as a means of assessing multiple aspects of acute MI care. **Indicator (Numerator):** Intrahospital mortality of patients with principal discharge diagnosis of acute myocardial infarction (MI), subcategorized by history of previous infarction, age, and intrahospital location of death.

CV-7

Indicator Focus: Diagnostic accuracy and resource utilization. **Indicator (Numerator):** Patients admitted for acute myocardial infarction (MI), rule-out acute MI, or unstable angina who have a discharge diagnosis of acute MI, subcategorized by admission to an intensive care unit, a monitored bed, or an unmonitored bed.

CHF Patient Population: Patients with a principal discharge diagnosis of congestive heart failure, with or without specific etiologies.

CV-8

Indicator Focus: Diagnostic accuracy. **Indicator (Numerator):** Patients with principal discharge diagnosis of congestive heart failure (CHF) with documented etiology and chest X-ray substantiation of CHF.

CV-9

Indicator Focus: Monitoring patient's response to therapy. **Indicator (Numerator):** Patients with a principal discharge diagnosis of congestive heart failure (CHF) and with at least two determinations of patient weight and of serum sodium, potassium, blood urea nitrogen (BUN), and creatinine levels.

TRAUMA Indicators for Beta Testing

Trauma Indicator Patient Population: Patients with ICD-9-CM diagnostic code of 800 through 959.9 who are either admitted to the hospital, die in the emergency department (ED), or are transferred from the hospital or the ED to another acute care facility, excluding patients with the following isolated injuries: burns; hip fractures in the elderly; specified fractures of the face, hand, and foot; and specified eye wounds.

TR-1

Indicator Focus: Efficiency of emergency medical services (EMS). **Indicator (Numerator):** Trauma patients with prehospital emergency medical services (EMS) scene time greater than 20 minutes.

TR-2

Indicator Focus: Ongoing monitoring of trauma patients. **Indicator (Numerator):** Trauma patients with blood pressure, pulse, respiration, and Glasgow Coma Scale (GCS) score documented in the emergency department (ED) record on arrival and hourly until inpatient admission to operating room or intensive care unit, death, or transfer to another care facility (hourly GCS needed only if altered state of consciousness).

TR-3

Indicator Focus: Airway management of comatose trauma patients. **Indicator (Numerator):** Comatose patients discharged from the emergency department (ED) prior to the establishment of a mechanical airway.

TR-4

Indicator Focus: Timeliness of diagnostic testing. **Indicator (Numerator):** Trauma patients with diagnosis of intracranial injury and altered state of consciousness upon emergency department (ED) arrival receiving initial head computerized tomography (CT) scan greater than 2 hours after ED arrival.

TR-5

Indicator Focus: Timeliness of surgical intervention for adult head injury. **Indicator (Numerator):** Trauma patients with diagnosis of extradural or subdural brain hemorrhage undergoing craniotomy greater than 4 hours after emergency department (ED) arrival (excluding intracranial pressure monitoring), subcategorized by pediatric or adult patients.

TR-6

Indicator Focus: Timeliness of surgical intervention for orthopedic injuries. **Indicator (Numerator):** Trauma patients with open fractures of the long bones as a result of blunt trauma receiving initial surgical treatment greater than 8 hours after emergency department (ED) arrival.

TR-7

Indicator Focus: Timeliness of surgical intervention for abdominal injuries. **Indicator (Numerator):** Trauma patients with diagnosis of laceration of the liver or spleen, requiring surgery undergoing laparotomy greater than 2 hours after emergency department (ED) arrival, subcategorized by pediatric or adult patients.

TR-8

Indicator Focus: Surgical decision making for abdominal gunshot and/or stab wounds. **Indicator (Numerator):** Trauma patients undergoing laparotomy for wounds penetrating the abdominal wall, subcategorized by gunshot and/or stab wounds.

TR-9

Indicator Focus: Timeliness of patient transfers. **Indicator (Numerator):** Trauma patients transferred from initial receiving hospital to another acute care facility within 6 hours from emergency department (ED) arrival to ED departure.

TR-10

Indicator Focus: Surgical decision making for orthopedic injuries. **Indicator (Numerator):** Adult trauma patients with femoral diaphyseal fractures treated by a nonfixation technique.

TR-11

Indicator Focus: Clinical decision making for potentially preventable deaths. **Indicator (Numerator):** Intrahospital mortality of trauma patients with one or more of the following conditions who did not undergo a procedure for the condition: tension pneumothorax, hemoperitoneum, hemothoraces, ruptured aorta, pericardial tamponade, and epidural of subdural hemorrhage.

TR-12

Indicator Focus: Systems necessary for obtaining autopsies for trauma victims. **Indicator (Numerator):** Trauma patients who expired within 48 hours of emergency department (ED) arrival for whom an autopsy was performed.

INFECTION CONTROL Indicators for Beta Testing

IC-1

Indicator Focus: Surgical wound infection. **Indicator (Numerator):** Selected inpatient and outpatient surgical procedures complicated by a wound infection during hospitalization or postdischarge.

IC-2

Indicator Focus: Postoperative pneumonia. **Indicator (Numerator):** Selected inpatient surgical procedures complicated by the onset of pneumonia during hospitalization but not beyond 10 postoperative days.

IC-3
Indicator Focus: Urinary catheter usage. **Indicator (Numerator):** Selected surgical procedures on inpatients who are catheterized during the perioperative period.

IC-4
Indicator Focus: Ventilator pneumonia. **Indicator (Numerator):** Ventilated patients who develop pneumonia.

IC-5
Indicator Focus: Postpartum endometritis. **Indicator (Numerator):** Inpatients who develop endometritis following cesarean section, followed until discharge.

IC-6
Indicator Focus: Concurrent surveillance of primary bloodstream infection. **Indicator (Numerator):** Inpatients with a central or umbilical line who develop primary bloodstream infection.

IC-7
Indicator Focus: Medical record abstraction of primary bloodstream infection. **Indicator (Numerator):** Inpatients with a central or umbilical line and primary bloodstream infection, analyzed by method of identification.

IC-8
Indicator Focus: Employee health program. **Indicator (Numerator):** Hospital staff who have been immunized for measles (rubeola) or are known to be immune.

MEDICATION USE Indicators for Beta Testing

MU-1
Indicator Focus: Individualizing dosage. **Indicator (Numerator):** Inpatients over 65 years old in whom creatinine clearance has been estimated.

MU-2

Indicator Focus: Individualizing dosage. **Indicator (Numerator):** Inpatients receiving parenteral aminoglycosides who have a measured aminoglycoside serum level.

MU-3

Indicator Focus: Reviewing the order. **Indicator (Numerator):** New medication orders prompting consultation by the pharmacist with physician or nurse subcategorized by orders changed.

MU-4

Indicator Focus: Timing of medication administration. **Indicator (Numerator):** Patients receiving intravenous prophylactic antibiotics within 2 hours before the first surgical incision.

MU-5

Indicator Focus: Accuracy of medication dispensing and administration. **Indicator (Numerator):** Number of reported significant medication errors.

MU-6

Indicator Focus: Informing the patient about the medication. **Indicator (Numerator):** Inpatients with principal and/or other diagnoses of insulin dependent diabetes mellitus who demonstrate self-blood glucose monitoring and self-administration of insulin before discharge, or are referred for postdischarge follow-up for diabetes management.

MU-7

Indicator Focus: Monitoring patient response. **Indicator (Numerator):** Inpatients receiving digoxin, theophylline, phenytoin, or lithium who have no corresponding measured drug levels or whose highest measured level exceeds a specific limit.

MU-8

Indicator Focus: Monitoring patient response. **Indicator (Numerator):** Inpatients receiving warfarin or intravenous therapeutic heparin who also receive vitamin K, protamine sulfate, or fresh frozen plasma.

MU-9

Indicator Focus: Reporting adverse drug reactions. **Indicator (Numerator):** ADRs reported through the hospital's ADR reporting system analyzed by method of reporting (spontaneous or retrospective medical record abstraction), type of ADR (dose related or nondose related), and time of occurrence (before admission or during hospitalization).

MU-10

Indicator Focus: Reviewing complete drug regimen. **Indicator (Numerator):** Inpatients receiving more than one type of oral benzodiazepine simultaneously.

MU-11

Indicator Focus: Reviewing complete drug regimen. **Indicator (Numerator):** Inpatients with seven or more prescribed medications on discharge.

MU-12

Indicator Focus: Overall performance of medication use system. **Indicator (Numerator):** Patients less than 25 years old with a principal discharge diagnosis of bronchoconstrictive pulmonary disease, who are readmitted to the hospital or visit the emergency department within 15 days of discharge due to an exacerbation of their principal diagnosis.

HOME INFUSION THERAPY Indicators for Beta Testing

IT-1

Indicator Focus: Unscheduled inpatient admission by type of therapy. **Indicator (Numerator):** Clients receiving home infusion therapy who have an unscheduled inpatient admission subcategorized by reason for admission.

IT-2

Indicator Focus: Discontinued infusion therapy by type of therapy. **Indicator (Numerator):** Courses of infusion therapy discontinued before prescribed completion, subcategorized by reason for discontinuation.

IT-3

Indicator Focus: Interruption in infusion therapy by type of therapy. **Indicator (Numerator):** Total number of interruptions in infusion therapy subcategorized by reason for interruption in therapy.

IT-4

Indicator Focus: Prevention and surveillance of infection by type of therapy. **Indicator (Numerator):** Clients with central lines whose catheter is removed or who receive antibiotic therapy for a confirmed or suspected catheter-related infection subcategorized by the type of central line catheter and number of lumens.

IT-5

Indicator Focus: Reporting adverse drug reactions. **Indicator (Numerator):** Total number of suspected or confirmed adverse drug reactions (ADRs) experienced by infusion therapy clients, subcategorized by the type and severity of ADR and by drug class.

IT-6

Indicator Focus: Client monitoring and appropriate intervention. **Indicator (Numerator):** Clients receiving total parenteral nutrition (TPN) and/or enteral therapy who are achieving or maintaining desired weight.

APPENDIX B

Joint Commission's Indicator Measurement System Performance Measures

---

1. **Focus:** Preoperative patient evaluation, intraoperative monitoring, and timely clinical intervention.
    Numerator: Patients developing a central nervous system (CNS) complication within two postprocedure days of procedures involving anesthesia* administration.

2. **Focus:** Preoperative patient evaluation, appropriate surgical preparation, intraoperative and postoperative monitoring, and timely clinical intervention.
    Numerator: Patients developing a peripheral neurological deficit within two postprocedure days of procedures involving anesthesia* administration.

3. **Focus:** Preoperative patient evaluation, intraoperative and postoperative monitoring, and timely clinical intervention.
    Numerator: Patients developing an acute myocardial infarction within two postprocedure days of procedures involving anesthesia* administration.

---

*For the indicators related to perioperative care, the population of interest includes all patients undergoing procedures involving anesthesia and an inpatient stay.

4.   **Focus:** Preoperative patient evaluation, intraoperative and postoperative monitoring, and timely clinical intervention.
     Numerator: Patients with a cardiac arrest within two postprocedure days of procedures involving anesthesia* administration.

5.   **Focus:** Preoperative patient evaluation, intraoperative and postoperative monitoring, and timely clinical intervention.
     Numerator: Intrahospital mortality of patients within two postprocedure days of procedures involving anesthesia* administration.

6.   **Focus:** Prenatal patient evaluation, education, and treatment selection.
     Numerator: Patients delivered by cesarean section.
     Denominator: All deliveries.

7.   **Focus:** Prenatal patient evaluation, education, and treatment selection.
     Numerator: Patients with vaginal birth after cesarean section (VBAC).
     Denominator: Patients delivered with a history of previous cesarean section.

8.   **Focus:** Prenatal patient evaluation, intrapartum monitoring, and clinical intervention.
     Numerator: Live-born infants with a birthweight less than 2,500 grams.
     Denominator: All live births.

9.   **Focus:** Prenatal patient evaluation, intrapartum monitoring, and clinical intervention.
     Numerator: Live-born infants with a birthweight greater than or equal to 2,500 grams, who have at least one of the

---

*For the indicators related to perioperative care, the population of interest includes all patients undergoing procedures involving anesthesia and an inpatient stay.

following: an Apgar score of less than 4 at five minutes, a requirement for admission to the neonatal intensive care unit within one day of delivery for greater than 24 hours, a clinically apparent seizure, or significant birth trauma.

Denominator: All live-born infants with a birthweight greater than 2,500 grams.

10. **Focus:** Prenatal patient evaluation, intrapartum monitoring, neonatal patient evaluation, and clinical intervention.

    Numerator: Live-born infants with a birthweight greater than 1,000 grams and less than 2,500 grams who have an Apgar score of less than 4 at five minutes.

    Denominator: All live-born infants with a birthweight greater than 1,000 grams and less than 2,500 grams.

11. **Focus:** Extended postoperative stay as a means of assessing multiple aspects of coronary artery bypass graft (CABG) care.

    Indicator Statement:* Patients undergoing isolated coronary artery bypass graft (CABG) procedures: number of days from initial surgery to discharge.

12. **Focus:** Timing of thrombolytic therapy administration.

    Indicator Statement: Patients admitted through the emergency department with a principal discharge diagnosis of acute myocardial infarction (AMI) receiving thrombolytic therapy: time from emergency department arrival to administration of thrombolytic therapy.

13. **Focus:** Diagnostic accuracy.

    Numerator: Patients with a principal discharge diagnosis of congestive heart failure with documented etiology.

    Denominator: Patients with a principal discharge diagnosis of congestive heart failure.

---

* An Indicator Statement (as contrasted with a numerator) is used when the measure is a continuous variable.

14. **Focus:** Extended postprocedure stay as a means of assessing multiple aspects of percutaneous transluminal coronary angioplasty (PTCA) care.

    Indicator Statement: Patients undergoing a percutaneous transluminal coronary angioplasty (PTCA): number of days from procedure to discharge.

15a. **Focus:** Intrahospital mortality as a means of assessing multiple aspects of coronary artery bypass graft (CABG) patient care.

    Numerator: Intrahospital mortality of patients undergoing an isolated CABG.

    Denominator: Patients undergoing an isolated CABG.

15b. **Focus:** Intrahospital mortality as a means of assessing multiple aspects of percutaneous transluminal coronary angioplasty (PTCA) patient care.

    Numerator: Intrahospital mortality of patients undergoing a PTCA.

    Denominator: Patients undergoing a PTCA.

15c. **Focus:** Intrahospital mortality as a means of assessing multiple aspects of acute myocardial infarction (AMI) patient care.

    Numerator: Intrahospital mortality of patients with a principal discharge diagnosis of acute myocardial infarction.

    Denominator: Patients with a principal discharge diagnosis of acute myocardial infarction.

16. **Focus:** Availability of data for diagnosis and staging.

    Numerator: Patients undergoing resection for primary cancer of the female breast, lung or colon/rectum for whom a surgical pathology consultation report is present in the medical record.

    Denominator: Patients undergoing resection for primary cancer of the female breast, lung, or colon/rectum.

17. **Focus:** Use of staging by managing physicians.

    Numerator: Patients undergoing resection for primary cancer of the female breast, lung, or colon/rectum with stage of tumor designated by a managing physician.

Denominator: Patients undergoing resection for primary cancer of the female breast, lung, or colon/rectum.

18. **Focus:** Use of tests critical for prognosis and clinical management of female breast cancer.

Numerator: Female patients with Stage I or greater primary breast cancer who, after initial biopsy or resection, have estrogen receptor analysis results in the medical record.

Denominator: Female patients with Stage I or greater primary breast cancer undergoing initial biopsy or resection.

19. **Focus:** Effectiveness of preoperative diagnosis and staging.

Numerator: Patients with non-small cell primary lung cancer undergoing thoracotomy with complete surgical resection of tumor.

Denominator: Patients with non-small cell primary lung cancer undergoing thoracotomy.

20. **Focus:** Comprehensiveness of diagnostic workup.

Numerator: Patients undergoing resection for primary cancer of the colon/rectum whose preoperative evaluation, by a managing physician, included examination of the entire colon.

Denominator: Patients undergoing resection for primary cancer of the colon/rectum.

21a. **Focus:** Ongoing monitoring of trauma patients.

Numerator: Trauma patients with systolic blood pressure, pulse rate, and respiratory rate documented on arrival to the emergency department (ED) and at least hourly for three hours or until ED disposition, whichever is earlier.

Denominator: All trauma patients.

21b. **Focus:** Ongoing monitoring of trauma patients.

Numerator: Trauma patients with selected intracranial injuries with Glasgow Coma Scale (GCS) score documented on arrival to emergency department (ED) and at least hourly for three hours or until ED disposition, whichever is earlier.

Denominator: Trauma patients with selected intracranial injuries.

22. **Focus:** Airway management of comatose trauma patients.

    Numerator: Comatose trauma patients with selected intracranial injuries discharged from the emergency department prior to endotracheal intubation or cricothyrotomy.

    Denominator: Emergency department comatose trauma patients with selected intracranial injuries.

23. **Focus:** Timeliness of diagnostic testing.

    Indicator Statement: Trauma patients with head computerized tomography (CT) scan performed: time from emergency department arrival to initial CT scan.

24a. **Focus:** Timeliness of surgical intervention for selected head injuries.

    Indicator Statement: Trauma patients undergoing selected neurosurgical procedures: time from emergency department arrival to procedure.

24b. **Focus:** Timeliness of intervention for selected orthopedic injuries.

    Indicator Statement: Trauma patients undergoing selected orthopedic procedures: time from emergency department arrival to procedure.

24c. **Focus:** Timeliness of surgical intervention for selected abdominal injuries.

    Indicator Statement: Trauma patients undergoing selected abdominal surgical procedures: time from emergency department arrival to procedure.

25a. **Focus:** Clinical decision making for potentially preventable deaths.

    Numerator: Intrahospital mortality of trauma patients with a diagnosis of pneumothorax or hemothorax who did not undergo a thoracostomy or thoracotomy.

Denominator: Intrahospital mortality of trauma patients with a diagnosis of pneumothorax or hemothorax.

25b. **Focus:** Clinical decision making for potentially preventable deaths.

Numerator: Intrahospital mortality of trauma patients with a systolic blood pressure of less than 70 mm Hg within two hours of emergency department arrival who did not undergo a laparotomy or thoracotomy.

Denominator: Intrahospital mortality of trauma patients with a systolic blood pressure of less than 70 mm Hg within two hours of emergency department arrival.

For Inclusion in 1996

26. **Focus:** Individualizing dosage.

Numerator: Inpatients 65 years of age or older in whom creatinine clearance has been estimated or measured.

Denominator: Inpatients 65 years of age or older.

27. **Focus:** Timing of medication administration.

Indicator Statement: Patient with selected surgical procedures receiving intravenous prophylactic antibiotics: timing of prophylactic antibiotic administration.

28. **Focus:** Informing the patient about the medication.

Numerator: Inpatients with a discharge diagnosis of insulin-dependent diabetes mellitus who demonstrate self-blood glucose monitoring and self-administration of insulin before discharge, or are referred for postdischarge follow-up for diabetes management.

Denominator: Inpatients with a discharge diagnosis of insulin-dependent diabetes mellitus.

29a. **Focus:** Monitoring patient response.

Numerator: Inpatients receiving digoxin who have no

corresponding measured drug level or whose highest measured level exceeds a specific limit.

Denominator: Inpatients receiving digoxin.

29b. Focus: Monitoring patient response.

Numerator: Inpatients receiving theophylline who have no corresponding measured drug level or whose highest measured level exceeds a specific limit.

Denominator: Inpatients receiving theophylline.

29c. Focus: Monitoring patient response.

Numerator: Inpatients receiving phenytoin who have no corresponding measured drug level or whose highest measured level exceeds a specific limit.

Denominator: Inpatients receiving phenytoin.

29d. Focus: Monitoring patient response.

Numerator: Inpatients receiving lithium who have no corresponding measured drug level or whose highest measured level exceeds a specific limit.

Denominator: Inpatients receiving lithium.

30. Focus: Reviewing complete drug regimen.

Indicator Statement: Inpatients: number of prescribed medications at discharge.

31. Focus: Surgical site infection.

Numerator: Selected inpatient and outpatient surgical procedures complicated by a surgical site infection.

Denominator: Number of selected inpatient and outpatient surgical procedures.

32. Focus: Ventilator-associated pneumonia.

Numerator: Ventilated inpatients who develop pneumonia.

Denominator: Inpatient ventilator days.

33. Focus: Surveillance of primary bloodstream infection.

Numerator: Inpatients with a central or umbilical line who develop primary bloodstream infection.

Denominator: Inpatient central or umbilical line days.

GLOSSARY OF TERMS

A

acceptability An overall assessment of care made by an individual or group. It is usually based on many dimensions of care including, but not limited to, its cost, appropriateness, availability, and effectiveness.

accessibility A performance dimension addressing the degree to which an individual or a defined population can approach, enter, and make use of needed health services. *See also* dimensions of performance.

accountability The obligation to disclose periodically, in adequate detail and consistent form, to all directly and indirectly responsible or properly interested parties, the purposes, principles, procedures, relationships, results, incomes, and expenditures involved in any activity, enterprise, or assignment so that they can be evaluated by the interested parties.

algorithm An ordered sequence of steps or instructions, with each step or instruction depending on the outcome of the previous one, that is used to tell how to solve a particular problem. An algorithm is specified exactly, so there can be no doubt about what to do next, and it has a finite number of steps. *See also* flowchart; indicator algorithm.

algorithm, indicator *See* indicator algorithm.

alpha-testing phase for indicator development The period of time in which Joint Commission indicators are tested in the field by voluntary accredited hospitals to clarify indicator definitions, eliminate certain indicators, and refine or modify other indicators. *See also* beta-testing phase for indicator development; post-beta-testing phase for indicator development.

appropriateness A performance dimension addressing the degree to which the care or intervention provided is relevant to a patient's clinical needs, given the current state of knowledge. *See also* dimensions of performance.

assessment The process of determining the value, significance, or extent of something, as in data assessment (determining the significance of data) or quality assessment (determining the extent to which quality is present). *See also* performance assessment.

assessment, performance *See* performance assessment.

assignable cause *See* special cause.

assignable-cause variation *See* special-cause variation.

attribute data Data that arise from the classification of items into categories; from counts of the number of items in a given category or the proportion in a given category; and from counts of the number of occurrences per unit. Attribute data can be arranged into naturally occurring or arbitrarily selected groups or sets of values, as opposed to continuous data, which have no naturally occurring breaks. An example of attribute data is the number of medical records that are complete and incomplete per given measurement period. Synonym: discrete data. *Compare* continuous data. *See also* data.

availability A performance dimension addressing the degree to which the care or intervention is performed when required by a patient. It is a measure of the supply of health resources and services relative to the needs or demands of an individual or a community. Health care is available when it can be obtained from appropriate personnel at the time and place it is needed.

Availability is a function of the distribution of appropriate resources and services and the willingness of the provider to render services to particular patients in need. *See also* dimensions of performance.

average value *See* location.

B

bell-shaped curve *See* normal distribution.

beta-testing phase for indicator development A period of time in which Joint Commission indicators are tested in the field by voluntary accredited hospitals. This testing phase is designed to evaluate the capacity of a wide variety of hospitals to collect and transmit indicator data to the Joint Commission, the capability of the Joint Commission's information system to receive and analyze such data and provide timely feedback to hospitals, indicator reliability and validity, and how indicator data may be incorporated into the accreditation process. *See also* alpha-testing phase for indicator development; post-beta-testing phase for indicator development.

black box technology The use of an unknown clinical performance measurement system without understanding its inner workings.

brainstorming A process used to elicit a large number of ideas from a group of people who are encouraged to use their collective thinking power to generate ideas and unrestrained thoughts in a relatively short period of time.

C

cause-and-effect diagram A pictorial display drawn to represent the relationship between some "effect" and all the possible "causes" influencing it. Synonyms: cause-effect diagram; fishbone diagram; Ishikawa diagram.

center line   The line on a graph representing the average value of the items being plotted. *See also* mean; median.

central tendency   *See* location.

chart, control   *See* control chart.

chart, run   *See* run chart.

checksheet   A data collection form that helps to summarize data based on sample observations and begin to identify patterns. A checksheet is used to answer the question, "How often are certain events happening?" It starts the process of translating opinions into facts. The completed form displays the data in a simple graphic summary. *See also* Pareto diagram.

clinical performance data   Neutral quantitative measurements of important patient care process or patient health outcomes, generated through application of performance measures commonly known as indicators; the output of performance measurement activities, and the input for the interpretive process. *See also* clinical performance information; data; performance.

clinical performance information   Clinical performance data that have been transformed through interpretation into a form useful for drawing conclusions and making decisions. *See also* clinical performance data; information; performance.

clinical relevance   *See* data relevance.

cognitive   Pertaining to the mental process or faculty of knowing, including awareness, perception, reasoning, and judgment. *See also* reason.

common cause   An ever-present factor that contributes to the random variation inherent in all processes. Common causes of variation are endogenous to a system and are not disturbances (they *are* the system) and can be removed or eliminated only by making basic changes in the system. *Synonyms:* endogenous cause; systemic cause. *See also* common-cause variation.

common-cause variation Fluctuation in a series of results that is due to the process and is produced by interactions of variables of that process. It is inherent in all processes. *Synonyms:* endogenous-cause variation; stable variation; systemic-cause variation. *See also* common cause; special-cause variation; variation.

communication The act of exchanging thoughts, messages, or information, as by speech, signals, writing, or behavior.

comparison The process of measuring and/or judging with the intent of determining the degree to which two or more objects of interest being compared are similar and different and by how much. *See also* comparison chart.

comparison chart A visual device used to study variation across different entities, such as the indicator rates among organizations reporting clinical performance data to a common performance database.

conclusion 1. Result or outcome of an act or process. 2. A judgment or decision reached after deliberation. *See also* summarizing data.

construct validity The degree to which a performance measure and its data quantify what they were designed to quantify. Construct validity that has been established for a measure or its data may be used as a criterion standard (gold standard) against which other measures are evaluated. *See also* convergent validity; data validity; scientific validity; validity.

continuity A performance dimension addressing the degree to which the care or intervention for a patient is coordinated among practitioners, among organizations, and over time. *See also* dimensions of performance.

continuous data   Data with a potentially infinite number of possible values along a continuum. An example of continuous data is the number of pounds a patient who is receiving total parenteral nutrition weighs over time or the number of minutes spent by prehospital personnel at a prehospital trauma scene. *Compare* attribute data. *See also* continuous variable; data.

continuous variable   A variable that, when measured, has a potentially infinite number of possible values along a continuum. *See also* continuous data; discrete variable.

control chart   A graphic display of data in the order that they occur with statistically determined upper and lower limits of expected common-cause variation. A control chart is used to indicate special causes of variation, to monitor a process for maintenance, and to determine if process changes have had the desired effect. *Compare* run chart. *See also* common-cause variation; control limit; special-cause variation; variation.

control limit   An expected limit of common-cause variation, sometimes referred to as either an upper or a lower control limit. Variation beyond a control limit is evidence that special causes are affecting a process or an outcome. *See also* common-cause variation; control chart; special cause.

convergent validity   Correlations among two or more measures, such as indicators or their data, of a concept. Convergent validity does not presuppose that one measure is a standard against which other measures should be evaluated. *See also* construct validity; data validity; scientific validity; validity.

curve, bell-shaped   *See* bell-shaped curve.

D

data The collection of material or facts on which a discussion or an inference is based, such as clinical performance data. Data are the product of measurement. *See also* attribute data; continuous data; clinical performance data; measurement.

data, attribute *See* attribute data.

data, clinical performance *See* clinical performance data.

data, continuous *See* continuous data.

data, discrete *See* attribute data.

data relevance One component of clinical performance data strength consisting of the degree to which clinical performance data identify real opportunities to improve processes and outcomes within an organization. Data that address irrelevant clinical issues will not be useful in decision making. *See also* data strength.

data reliability The extent to which data results are consistent across repeated measurements of the same phenomenon by different measurers or at different times by the same measurers. The phenomenon must not have changed in the interval between measurements. *See also* data; reliability.

data set, indicator *See* indicator data set.

data significance *See* data relevance.

data strength The degree to which data demonstrate six important attributes: clinical relevance, range of health care processes and outcomes addressed, reliability, validity, variation, and provider control. *See also* data relevance.

data summary *See* summarizing data.

data validity The extent to which data measure only what they were intended to measure. *See also* data; validity.

dependent variable A variable whose value is dependent on the effect of independent variable(s) in the relationship under study. In statistics, the dependent variable is the one predicted by a regression equation. *Compare* independent variable. *See also* variable.

desirable outcome An outcome that is recommendable or advisable; for example, survival following an intervention is a desirable outcome. *See also* outcome; undesirable outcome.

desirable process A process that is recommendable or advisable; for example, timely monitoring of vital signs of seriously injured patients is a desirable process of care. *See also* process; undesirable process.

deviation, standard *See* standard deviation.

diagram, Pareto *See* Pareto diagram.

dimensions of performance Attributes of organizational performance that are related to organizations doing the "right things" (for example, appropriateness) and "doing things well" (for example, effectiveness). Performance dimensions are definable, measurable, and improvable. *See also* appropriateness; availability; continuity; effectiveness; efficacy; efficiency; respect and caring; safety; timeliness.

discrete data *See* attribute data.

discrete variable A measurement that is limited to discrete options; for example, yes/no/unknown. *See also* continuous variable.

dispersion *See* spread.

distribution *See* frequency distribution.

distribution, frequency *See* frequency distribution.

distribution, normal *See* normal distribution.

E

effectiveness A performance dimension addressing the degree to which the care or intervention is provided in the correct manner, given the current state of knowledge, in order to achieve the desired or projected outcome for a patient. Effectiveness is not synonymous with efficiency; a consideration of cost is not required. *See also* dimensions of performance.

efficacy 1. A performance dimension addressing the degree to which the care or intervention for a patient has been shown to accomplish the desired or projected outcome(s). 2. The extent to which a specific intervention, procedure, regimen, or service produces a beneficial result under ideal conditions. Efficacy is often used as a synonym for effectiveness in health care delivery. Efficacy is sometimes distinguished from effectiveness to mean the results of actions undertaken under ideal circumstances, with the term "effectiveness" meaning the results of actions under usual or normal circumstances. *See also* dimensions of performance.

efficiency A performance dimension addressing the relationship between the outcomes (results of the care or intervention) and the resources used to deliver the care or intervention. The ultimate measure of efficiency is the cost of achieving a goal to the benefit achieved by the goal. *See also* dimensions of performance.

endogenous cause *See* common cause.

endogenous-cause variation *See* common-cause variation.

error, random *See* random error.

exogenous cause *See* special cause.

exogenous-cause variation *See* special-cause variation.

explicit approach to interpretation An approach characterized by clearly developed, expressly stated, and carefully delineated tasks. *See also* interpretation; rational approach to interpretation; thesis of interpretation.

extrasystemic cause *See* special cause.

extrasystemic-cause variation *See* special-cause variation.

F

fishbone diagram *See* cause-and-effect diagram.

flowchart A pictorial summary that shows with symbols and words the steps, sequence, and relationship of the various operations involved in the performance of a function or a process. A flowchart describes an algorithm. Synonym: flow diagram. *See also* algorithm.

frequency distribution In statistics, the complete summary of the frequencies of the values or categories of measurement made on a group of persons or other entities. The distribution tells either how many or what proportion of the group was found to have each value (or each range of values) out of all the possible values that the quantitative measure can have. A bell-shaped curve or normal distribution is an example of a distribution in which the greatest number of observations fall in the center with fewer and fewer observations falling evenly on either side of the average. Synonym: distribution. *See also* interquartile range; location; mean; median; mode; range; spread; standard deviation.

G

GCS *See* Glasgow Coma Scale.

Glasgow Coma Scale (GCS) In trauma care, a scoring instrument used to quantify depth and duration of impaired consciousness based on a patient's eye opening, verbal performance, and motor responsiveness. The GCS was developed to allow for reliable assessment and recording of changing states of altered neurological status over time. The 15-point scale demonstrates better neurological function with higher numbers. It has limited utility in estimating prognosis or outcome.

H

high cost Processes or outcomes for which total expenses are elevated by one of two criteria: either the absolute cost or the cost compared to some point. *See also* high risk; high visibility; high volume; problem prone.

high risk 1. Three categories of patient care processes: processes that are needed but not performed; "risky" processes that are performed but not needed; and processes that are needed and performed, but performed poorly. 2. Processes that are inherently risky because the services being provided may never have been performed before or have been performed so few times that their safety and efficacy remain under investigation. 3. Processes that are performed for patients whose preexisting characteristics may adversely influence the outcomes. *See also* high cost; high visibility; high volume; problem prone.

high visibility Processes or outcomes thrust into the limelight by the media. *See also* high cost; high risk; high volume; problem prone.

high volume Patient care processes that are performed frequently, affect large numbers of patients, or both; patient health outcomes that occur frequently, affect large numbers of patients, or both. *See also* high cost; high risk; high visibility; problem prone.

I

improvement, performance *See* performance improvement.

IMS *See* Indicator Measurement System.

IMSystem *See* Indicator Measurement System.

independent variable The characteristic being observed or measured that is hypothesized to influence an event or manifestation (the dependent variable) within the defined area of the relationships under study. The independent variable is not influenced by the event or manifestation but may cause it or contribute to its variation. In statistics, an independent variable is one of several variables that appear as arguments in a regression equation. *Compare* dependent variable. *See also* variable.

indicator A measure used to quantify and improve performance of functions, processes, and outcomes. *See also* performance measure.

indicator algorithm An ordered sequence of data element retrieval and aggregation through which numerator events and denominator events are identified by an indicator. Synonym: indicator data collection logic. *See also* algorithm; indicator.

indicator data set A collection of clinical performance data generated by a single indicator that was developed to frame and quantify an important dimension of a particular performance issue; a specific data focus. *See also* clinical performance data; indicator.

indicator development, alpha-testing phase for *See* alpha-testing phase for indicator development.

indicator development, beta-testing phase for *See* beta-testing phase for indicator development.

indicator development, post-beta-testing phase for *See* post-beta-testing phase for indicator development.

indicator information set Indicator-specific information typically composed of an indicator statement, definition of terms, indicator type, rationale, description of indicator population, indicator data collection logic, and underlying causes that may explain undesirable variation in data; provides users with the important characteristics of indicator data. *See also* indicator.

Indicator Measurement System (IMSystem, IMS) A performance measurement system developed by the Joint Commission in conjunction with accredited health care organizations. It is designed to 1. continuously collect objective performance data that are derived from the application of aggregate data indicators by heath care organizations; 2. aggregate, risk-adjust as necessary, and analyze the performance data on a national level; 3. provide comparative data to participating organizations for use in their internal performance improvement efforts; 4. identify patterns that may call for more focused attention by the Joint Commission at the organizational level; and 5. provide a national performance database that can serve as a resource for health services research. Formerly (1992) indicator monitoring system.

information Data that have been transformed through analysis and interpretation into a form useful for drawing conclusions and making decisions. *See also* conclusion; data.

information set, indicator *See* indicator information set.

innumeracy The inability to express oneself in quantitative terms. *Compare* numeracy.

inspection 1. The process of examining carefully. 2. Activities, such as measuring, examining, testing, gauging one or more characteristics of a product or service and comparing these with specified requirements to determine conformity. Inspection is a past-oriented strategy that attempts to identify unacceptable output after it has been produced and separate it from the good output.

interpretation The multistep process by which meaning is assigned to raw clinical performance data; the process of making sense of, or understanding data. *See also* explicit approach to interpretation; rational approach to interpretation; thesis of interpretation.

interpretation, rational approach to   *See* rational approach to interpretation.

interpretation, thesis of   *See* thesis of interpretation.

interquartile range   A measure of spread around the median of a distribution. The interquartile range and median are well suited for non-normal frequency distributions. *See also* frequency distribution; median; spread.

Ishikawa diagram   *See* cause-and-effect diagram.

L

location   In statistics, a measure of the position of a frequency distribution. *Synonyms:* central tendency; average value. *See also* frequency distribution; spread.

lower control limit   *See* control limit.

M

mean   A measure of central tendency of a collection of data specifying the arithmetic average. A mean consists of all the measurements of the data set divided by the total number of measurements in the data set. The mean is best used when the distribution of data is balanced and unimodal. In a normal distribution, the mean coincides with the median and mode. *Synonym:* average. *Compare* median; mode. *See also* frequency distribution; normal distribution.

measurable   Possible to be quantified, as in measurable temperature or measurable performance. *See also* measurement.

measure   1. A quantitative tool or instrument used to make measurements. 2. A unit, such as an inch, specified by a measurement scale. 3. The act or process of measuring. *See also* measurement; performance measure.

measurement 1. The process of quantification, that is, determining that attribute of a thing by which it is greater or less than some other thing. *See also* performance measurement. 2. The number resulting from a quantification process. 3. Pertaining to the process of measurement, as in measurement data or measurement error.

measurement, performance *See* performance measurement.

Measurement System, Indicator *See* Indicator Measurement System.

measure, performance *See* performance measure.

median A measure of central tendency of a collection of data, consisting of the middle number of a data set when the measurements are arranged sequentially from smallest to largest or from largest to smallest. It is the most valid measure of central tendency whenever a distribution is skewed. *Compare* mean; mode. *See also* frequency distribution.

mode A measure of central tendency of a collection of data consisting of the measurement of the data set that occurs most often. *Compare* mean; median. *See also* frequency distribution.

N

normal distribution A frequency distribution in which the greatest number of observations fall in the center with fewer and fewer observations falling evenly on either side of the average. *Synonym:* bell-shaped curve. *See also* frequency distribution.

numeracy The ability to think and express oneself in quantitative terms. *Compare* innumeracy.

O

outcome The cumulative effect at a defined point in time of performing one or more processes in the care of a patient; for example, patient survival (or death) following a health intervention is an outcome. *See also* desirable outcome; undesirable outcome.

P

Pareto analysis   The application of the principle of determining which few steps in a process are vital or most important and taking action to alter or reinforce these steps, rather than the many other incidental steps in the process. *See also* Pareto diagram.

Pareto chart   *See* Pareto diagram.

Pareto diagram   A special form of vertical bar graph that displays information in such a way that priorities for process improvement can be established. It displays the relative importance of all the data and is used to direct efforts to the largest improvement opportunity by highlighting the vital few in contrast to the many others. *See also* Pareto analysis; Pareto principle.

Pareto principle   A principle that is employed to identify the "vital few" to help direct resources and attention to areas where they do the most good. The Pareto principle states that a few contributors to the cost of poor quality are responsible for the bulk of the cost. These vital few contributors need to be identified so that improvement resources can be concentrated in the few contributors. *See also* Pareto analysis.

performance   The way in which an individual, group, or organization carries out or accomplishes its important functions and processes; for example, measuring the performance of a health plan in providing obstetrical care of high quality. *See also* performance assessment; performance improvement; performance measure; performance measurement.

performance assessment   An analysis and interpretation of performance measurement data to transform them into useful information; the second segment of a performance measurement, assessment, and improvement system. The product of assessment is information. *See also* assessment; information; interpretation; performance; performance improvement.

performance data, clinical *See* clinical performance data.

performance, dimensions of *See* dimensions of performance.

performance improvement The study and adaptation of functions and processes to increase the probability of achieving desired outcomes; the third segment of a performance measurement, performance assessment, and performance improvement system.

performance measure Any instrument (such as an indicator) for quantifying levels of performance. *See also* indicator; measure; performance.

performance measurement The quantification of processes and outcomes using one or more dimensions of performance, such as timeliness or availability; the first segment of a performance measurement, performance assessment, and performance improvement system. *See also* dimensions of performance; measurement; performance.

post-beta-testing phase of indicator development A period of time following the beta-testing phase of indicator development in which data are analyzed according to specific criteria in order to finalize a set of indicators for inclusion in the Joint Commission's Indicator Measurement System (IMSystem). *See also* beta-testing phase for indicator development; Indicator Measurement System.

principle, Pareto *See* Pareto principle.

problem prone Processes that have produced problems for patients, their families, health care providers, and purchasers because organizational systems do not work. *See also* high cost; high risk; high visibility; high volume.

process An interrelated series of activities, actions, events, mechanisms, or steps that transform inputs into outputs for a particular beneficiary or customer. *See also* desirable process, undesirable process.

process, desirable *See* desirable process.

process variation The spread of process output over time. There is variation in every process, and all variation is caused. The causes are of two types: special and common. A process can have both types of variation at the same time or only common-cause variation. The management action necessary to improve the process is different depending on the type of variation being addressed. *See also* common-cause variation; special-cause variation; variation.

process, undesirable *See* undesirable process.

R

random error Error caused by chance factors that confound the measurement of processes and outcomes. The amount of random error is inversely related to an indicator's degree of reliability. The effects of random error are unsystematic. *See also* reliability.

range In a data set, the distance between the lowest and highest values. It is calculated by subtracting the lowest value in the data set from the highest value in the same set. Its usefulness as a measure of spread is limited because it is based on only the two extreme values in a data set and ignores the distribution of all the values within those limits. *Compare* standard deviation. *See also* frequency distribution; interquartile range; spread.

range, interquartile *See* interquartile range.

rational Exercising the ability to reason. *See also* rational approach to interpretation; reason.

rational approach to interpretation An approach characterized by use of informed reason, rather than emotion or personal prejudice, to form judgments. A rational approach to interpretation is important because individual subjective, or intuitive, judgments tend to be biased and inaccurate. *See also* interpretation; explicit approach to interpretation; rational; thesis of interpretation.

reason The capacity for logical, rational, and analytic thought; intelligence, good judgment, sound sense. *See also* cognitive.

regression In statistics, the relationship between the mean value of a random variable and the corresponding values of one or more independent variables. A common form of regression is a linear regression in which the model chosen for the analysis is a linear equation. *See also* regression analysis.

regression analysis A statistical procedure for determining the best approximation of the relationship between a dependent variable, such as the revenues of a hospital, and one or more independent variables, such as gross national product or per capita income. By measuring exactly how large and significant each independent variable has historically been in its relation to the dependent variable, the future value of the dependent variable can be predicted. Regression analysis attempts to measure the degree of correlation between dependent and independent variables, thereby establishing the predictive value of the independent variable. The most common form of regression analysis is a linear regression model. Multiple regression analysis is a method for measuring the effects of several factors concurrently. *See also* regression.

relevance, clinical *See* data relevance.

relevance, data *See* data relevance.

reliability 1. Consistency in results of a measure, including the tendency of the measure to produce the same results twice when it measures some entity or attribute believed not to have changed in the interval between measurements. 2. Statistically, the degree to which scores are free from random error. *See also* data reliability; random error.

reliability, data   *See* data reliability.

respect and caring   A performance dimension addressing the degree to which a patient, or a designee, is involved in his or her own care decisions and to which those providing services do so with sensitivity and respect for the patient's needs, expectations, and individual differences. *See also* dimensions of performance.

risk adjustment   A statistical method of analysis that attempts to control for bias due to confounding factors. Risk adjustment allows interpreters to estimate what would have happened if both comparison groups had been the same when, in fact, they were not. That is, the estimate of the difference between the two comparison groups is adjusted to compensate for the differences between the groups on the confounding factors, such as age.

risk management   In health care, the function of planning, organizing, and directing a comprehensive program of activities to identify, evaluate, and take corrective action against risks that may lead to patient injury, employee injury, and property loss or damage with resulting institutional financial loss or legal liability.

run chart   A display of performance data in which data points are plotted as they occur over time to detect trends or other patterns and variation occurring over time. Run charts cannot distinguish variation arising from common causes versus special causes. *Compare* control chart. *See also* data; variation.

S

safety   1. Freedom of danger, risk, or injury. 2. A performance dimension addressing the degree to which the risk of an intervention (for example, use of a drug or a procedure) and risk in the care environment are reduced for a patient and other persons, including health care practitioners. *See also* dimensions of performance.

scatter *See* spread.

scientific validity The degree to which a demonstrable, causal relationship exists between a process and the outcomes of the process. *See also* construct validity; convergent validity; data validity; validity.

special cause A factor that intermittently and unpredictably induces variation over and above that inherent in a system. It often appears as an extreme point, such as a point beyond the control limits on a control chart, or some specific, identifiable pattern in data. *Synonyms:* assignable cause; exogenous cause; extrasystemic cause. *See also* common cause; special-cause variation; variation.

special-cause variation Fluctuation in a series of results that is due to factors that intermittently and unpredictably induce variation over and above that inherent in a particular system. Special causes of variation are not part of the process or system all the time or do not affect everyone, but arise because of specific circumstances. Special-cause variation tends to cluster by person, place, and time, and should be eliminated by an organization if it results in undesirable outcomes. *Synonyms:* assignable-cause variation; exogenous-cause variation; extrasystemic-cause variation; unstable variation. *See also* common-cause variation; variation.

spread In statistics, a measure of the scatter around an average value. *Synonyms:* dispersion; scatter. *See also* frequency distribution; interquartile range; location; range; standard deviation.

stable variation *See* common-cause variation.

standard deviation A measure of a frequency distribution's spread that is equal to the square root of the mean of all the squares of the deviations from the mean. *Compare* interquartile range; range. *See also* frequency distribution; mean; spread.

summarizing data The process of expressing unsorted raw data in a form that will permit, directly or by means of further calculations, conclusions to be drawn. *See also* conclusion; data.

systemic cause *See* common cause.

systemic-cause variation *See* common-cause variation.

T

tampering Taking action on some signal of variation without taking into account the difference between special-cause and common-cause variation. *See also* variation.

thesis of interpretation The proposition that drawing accurate conclusions from raw clinical performance data depends on the degree to which the interpretive process is performed in an explicit and rational, or formal, manner.

timeliness A performance dimension addressing the degree to which the care or intervention is provided to a patient at the most beneficial or necessary time. *See also* dimensions of performance.

U

undesirable outcome An outcome that is not recommended or advised; for example, mortality following an intervention is an undesirable outcome. *See also* desirable outcome; outcome.

undesirable process A process that is not recommended or advised; for example, discharging comatose patients from the emergency department to inpatient destinations without a mechanical airway in place is an undesirable process. *See also* desirable process; process.

unstable variation *See* special-cause variation.

unusual variation A departure from steady-state variation, as in special-cause variation. *See also* special-cause variation; variation.

upper control limit *See* control limit.

V

validity 1. The degree to which an observed situation reflects the true situation. 2. In performance measurement, the degree to which an indicator or other measure identifies an event that merits further review by various individuals or groups providing or affecting the process or outcome defined by the indicator or other measure. *See also* construct validity; convergent validity; data validity; scientific validity.

validity, construct *See* construct validity.

validity, convergent *See* convergent validity.

validity, scientific *See* scientific validity.

validity, data *See* data validity.

variable 1. Any item, such as quantity, attribute, phenomenon, or event, that can have different values. Examples are length in millimeters, time in minutes, and temperature in degrees. *See also* dependent variable; independent variable. 2. Something that varies, as in a variable number of factors.

variable, continuous *See* continuous variable.

variable, dependent *See* dependent variable.

variable, discrete *See* discrete variable.

variable, independent *See* independent variable.

variation Fluctuation in a series of results. A certain amount of variation is the inevitable product (output) of any system or process.

Unusual variation is a departure from this steady state. *See also* common-cause variation; control chart; process variation; special-cause variation; tampering.

variation, common-cause   *See* common-cause variation.

variation, process   *See* process variation.

variation, special-cause   *See* special-cause variation.

variation, stable   *See* common-cause variation.

variation, unstable   *See* special-cause variation.

INDEX

flowcharts and, 32, 169–173
frequency distribution
and, 104
Pareto diagrams and, 29, 32,
182, 183–192
provider control and, 90
Undesirable processes/outcomes,
14, 48, 59–60, 238
provider control and, 90
relevance and, 69–71
Undesirable variation, 13, 21–22,
29, 127–165
data characteristics and, 63
provider control and
comparison charts and,
32, 161
underlying causes of. *See*
Underlying causes
Unpredictability, 71, 142
Unreliability, 74, 84, 93
Unstable variation, 21. *See also*
Special-cause variation
Unusual variation, 21, 32, 128–129,
239, 240

V

Validity, 5, 93
construct, 81–82, 221
convergent, 82, 222
data strength and, 15, 80–84
defined, 80, 94, 223, 239
indicator development and,
42, 45
scientific, 82, 237
testing, 82–84
types of, 81–82
Value
average, 21, 84, 87, 94
creation of, 21, 32

frequency distribution and, 97–
98. *See also* Frequency
distribution
outlier, 104, 106, 107
undesirable variation and,
21, 32
See also Mean; Median; Mode
Variability, 110–112, 125. *See also*
Dispersion
Variables
continuous versus discrete, 14,
48, 55–59, 115–116. *See*
also Continuous variable;
Discrete variable
data dredging and, 41
defined, 239
dependent, 224
independent, 228
Variables control chart, 58,
144–145
Variables data
confounding factors and, 156
control chart for, 144–145
Variance, 109–110, 158
Variation, 21
assessing, 84–88
characterizing, 127–128
common-cause versus special-
cause, 128, 131–139. *See*
also Common-cause
variation; Special-cause
variation
comparison chart and, 32, 153,
161
control chart and, 132, 147–152.
See also Control chart
data strength and, 15, 84–89
defined, 127, 239–240
degrees of, 86–87, 94